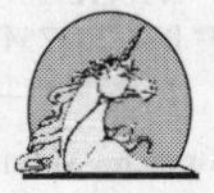

Sunita Pant Bansal

CHOLESTEROL BUSTERS

+ *A 15-Day Detox Plan to Reduce Cholesterol*

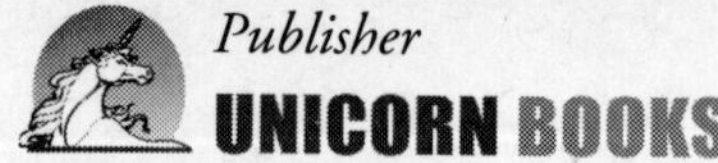

F-2/16, Ansari Road, Daryaganj, New Delhi-110002
☎ 011-23275434, 23262683, 23250704 • *Fax:* 011-23257790
E-mail: info@unicornbooks.in • *Website:* www.unicornbooks.in

Branch : Mumbai
23-25, Zaoba Wadi Thakurdwar, Mumbai-401002
☎ 022-22010941, 022-22053387
E-mail: rapidex@bom5.vsnl.net.in

Showroom :
★ **PM Publications,** New Delhi
- 10-B, Netaji Subhash Marg, Daryaganj
  New Delhi-110002
- 6686, Khari Baoli, Delhi-110006

Distributors :
★ **Pustak Mahal,** New Delhi
Delhi: ☎ 011-23276539
Bengaluru: ☎ 080-22234025
Patna: ☎ 0612-3294193

★ **V & S Publishers,** Hyderabad
☎ 040-24737290

ISBN 978-81-7806-107-4
Cholesterol Busters

Edition: 2012

***Printed at :** Unique Color Carton, Mayapuri, New Delhi-110064*

To my family

whose unflinching support

always makes me move ahead

without looking back.

Acknowledgement

Whenever I write any book on nutrition and health, I can not help but remember my father, who introduced this subject into my life. Today all my theories and statements can be traced back to him. I humbly acknowledge his blessings all through the research and writing of this book.

All credit for making me work on this particular topic goes to Dr Ashok Gupta, the publisher of this book. His faith in my work encourages me to continue finding time to write for him. I hope our brainstorming sessions would result in a few more of such useful titles for our readers.

Many thanks to my assistant, Sujith V.M., for typesetting my research material to give it the shape of a book.

–Sunita Pant Bansal

New Delhi, India

March, 2006

Contents

Introduction

Over the past couple of decades there has been a growing concern about cholesterol. Doctors have been telling us that fat is a killer. Eat less cholesterol, saturated fat and salt; eat more fibre rich foods we are told. If we do not, we are doomed to the West's greatest killer - heart disease, if not that, then stroke. A high cholesterol level in the blood is also related to an increased incidence of gallstones.

The most common life-threatening disease, which seems to be in our control, is the Heart Disease; Cancer and AIDS being out of bounds. There are many diseases that affect the heart, but the one that the 'healthy eating' strategies seek to prevent is Coronary Heart Disease (CHD) or Ischaemic Heart Disease (IHD). CHD is a condition where the coronary arteries that supply blood to nourish the heart muscle are narrowed by a build-up of material on their walls (an atheroma) to such an extent that they become blocked. This cuts off the blood supply to part of the heart muscle, and we have a heart attack. The narrowing also encourages the clotting of blood and, in consequence, it is possible for a clot to cause a heart attack long before the atheroma is large enough to do so. The clot may travel and if it reaches the brain and causes a blockage, it causes a stroke. The material generally found in the build-up is cholesterol and the 'healthy eating' advice given to people to reduce the incidence of CHD and stroke is aimed simply at reducing the levels of cholesterol in the blood.

High cholesterol in itself is not a disease, but a side-effect of an unhealthy lifestyle. The incidence of cholesterol related problems are on the increase, and diet alone can not be blamed for it; lack of exercise, choice of beverages, cigarette smoking, undisciplined work and social life also play a significant role in the cholesterol production in our body. The way to balance the cholesterol in the body, is to live like our fore-fathers for they walked a lot, were close to nature, ate the seasonal fruits and vegetables and lived a disciplined life.

Let us understand this whole thing systematically, so that we are able to look after ourselves better.

As dieticians we are taught the principles of diet-therapy according to certain fixed allopathic norms, as we are supposed to help the doctors in treating the disease. It certainly helps to understand the human anatomy and physiology, coupled with biochemistry, but somehow I always felt that it was (and still is) not complete. We saw the things through only one perspective, in the isolation of our laboratories. We looked at the symptoms and treated them in the fixed parameters of the human body as a machine. This superficial approach worked most of the time, but then sometimes it didn't.

That is when I started studying other alternative therapies, and found that all of them related all the diseases to nature, which is logical as we are part of and are affected by our environment. Any imbalance in nature and our immediate environment affects us. Certain effects are obvious, like dropping of body resistance during change of climate and thereby catching infections like influenza. But then there are other subtler environmental changes like a change in the job, or family environment (marriage, childbirth, death), which also affect our bodies (internally) and since any action results in a reaction, so our body also reacts. So without our knowledge, over years of absorption from our surroundings, we accumulate a lot of emotional and physiological toxins, which ultimately manifest as disease.

Production of cholesterol (among other things) is also one of our body's reactions towards stress. By simply reducing its intake through the diet and taking medicines to remove it, is again treating the problem symptomatically. This is not a permanent solution. The solution would be to understand the genesis of the problem, so that when you treat it, it does not recur.

After much study of the possible causes and various alternative therapies, I arrived at certain conclusions and devised a fifteen-day detox programme, which if followed regularly, yields positive results in six to eight weeks. It involves a regular intake of cholesterol-busting foods coupled with a healthy disciplined lifestyle regime. This simple programme breaks down the existing cholesterol deposits in the body, lowers the blood cholesterol levels and controls the further production of cholesterol by the body, bringing about a drastic upliftment in the physical and mental well-being of the person who makes a habit of it.

Part I

Our Food

Our food contains carbohydrates, proteins, vitamins, minerals and fats. Carbohydrates are energy giving, proteins are body building, vitamins and minerals maintain the health of the body and fats are pure concentrated sources of energy. Other than that, fats are an essential part of the structure of cell membranes and also play a role in the formation of various hormones in our body.

According to the nutrients they contribute, the various foods can be divided into seven groups.

- The first group consists of milk and its products. An adult requires 1-2 servings of milk or its products everyday, and a child needs to have a minimum of 2-3 servings of milk daily. Besides providing good quality protein, milk also gives us calcium (for bones and teeth) and vitamin B complex. An average serving would be: 180ml milk/ 200gm yoghurt/ 30gm cheese.

- The second group contains fats and oils (including butter, cream, *vanaspati, ghee,* etc.). The minimum daily fat/oil intake should be 3-tablespoons. This is chiefly the energy providing group.
- The third group is that of the cereals. These are valuable for protein, iron, B complex vitamins and calories. They provide roughage that allows easy bowel movement and keeps the digestive system in order. Items include various types of bread, *chapatis, idli, dosa,* macaroni, noodles, rice etc. Any of these should be taken in every major meal, that is six to seven servings (20gm per serving, raw) per day.
- The fourth group is that of proteins (body building) and contains meat, fish and poultry for non-vegetarians and nuts, *dals* and beans for the vegetarians. One to two servings (30gm per serving, raw) from this group is a must in our daily diet.
- The fifth group is a provider of vitamin A (for eyes) and iron (blood formation). This includes

all the green leafy vegetables like spinach, mint etc. Besides maintaining the health of eyes and the skin, these vegetables have roughage enough for regular elimination habits (bowel habits). Three or more servings (100gm per serving, raw) of this group are essential in our daily diet.

- ❖ The sixth group contains all the remaining vegetables and fruits. Two or more servings (100gm per serving, raw) of this group is also essential in our diet every day. This group is a provider of all the vitamins and minerals, which are essential for the normal functioning of our body system, which in turn is responsible for the healthy glow on our face, shine in our eyes and the health of our hair.

- ❖ The last group is an important group since it provides us with vitamin C. This vitamin is necessary for the health of our gums and blood vessels. Also it protects us from contracting any kind of infections, especially cold and cough. Vitamin C sources are all the citrus fruits like oranges and lemons, tomatoes, amla and guava. Even green chillies and capsicum are rich in vitamin C. A daily serving (50gm per serving, raw) of this group is desired. Since vitamin C is very sensitive to heat, it is suggested to eat the raw fruits/vegetables as much as possible.

Out of the above, there is no group which provides all the essential nutrients, that is why every group is necessary in our daily diet to maintain a balance among all the nutrients. Sugar is not part of any food group as it provides only calories and no other nutrients.

This sounds easy and we may believe that once we are having a balanced diet, there should be no possibility of any kind of disease (chronic diseases, as infections and accidents may be unavoidable) affecting us. But food plays a small role in sickness, as research has shown that our minds also have an important role to play in our state of health or disease. A stressed mind results in producing toxins in our body that may accumulate to manifest as a chronic disease. So once we have understood our diet, we should understand our mental stresses and try to get rid of them. In this way we would effectively be able to control our chronic diseases.

Average nutritive value of foods per 100g

Foodstuffs	*Proteins (g)*	*Fats (g)*	*Carbohydrates (g)*	*Calories (Kcal)*
All Cereals	9.9	2.3	71.0	344
Bread	7.8	0.7	51.9	245
Salty biscuit	6.6	32.4	54.6	534
Sweet biscuit	6.4	15.2	71.9	450
All Pulses	22.6	2.0	58.4	342
Green leafy vegetables	3.8	0.6	6.0	45
Roots and Tubers	1.2	0.2	16.0	70
Other vegetables	2.2	0.3	6.3	36
Nuts and Oilseeds	15.2	46.6	20.4	578
Condiments & Spices	9.8	6.6	40.6	261
Fruits	1.1	0.4	7.6	79
Meat	21.0	4.9	0.8	131
Egg	13.3	13.3	–	173
Milk	3.6	5.8	4.7	85
Curd (Yoghurt)	3.1	4.0	3.0	60
Butter	–	81.0	–	729
Ghee	- -	100.0	–	900
Oil	–	100.0	–	900
Sugar	0.1	- -	99.4	398
Honey	0.3	- -	79.5	319
Jaggery	0.4	0.1	95.0	383
Sago	0.2	0.2	87.1	351

Source: S. *Pasricha, Count What You Eat, NIN, Hyderabad,* 1989.

Fats in the Food

Our major concern in this book is the fat content of our diet, as cholesterol belongs to the family of fats. First of all we must understand what they are and the role they play in our health. Then we shall be able to decide how much we need them and what should be done to the excess that we may have accumulated unknowingly.

Fats in the food may be visible as in the form of *ghee*, butter, cream, oil; or invisible as present in whole milk, red meat, nuts and oilseeds.

Role of fat

Fat is one of the three nutrients (along with protein and carbohydrates) that supply calories to the body. Fat provides nine calories per gram, more than twice the number provided by carbohydrates or protein.

Fat is essential for the proper functioning of the body. Fats provide the 'essential' fatty acids, which are not made by the body and must be obtained from food. Linoleic acid is the most important essential fatty acid, especially for the growth and development of infants. Fatty acids provide the raw materials that help in the control of blood clotting, inflammation, and other body functions.

Fat serves as the storage substance for the body's extra calories. The adipose tissue thus formed helps insulate the body. Fats are also an important energy source. When the body has used up the calories from carbohydrates, which occurs after the first twenty minutes of exercise, it begins to utilise the calories from fat.

Healthy skin and hair are maintained by fat as it helps in the absorption, and transport through the bloodstream of the fat-soluble vitamins A, D, E, and K responsible for the health of skin, hair, eyes and bones.

Structure of fat

Fats are built of **fatty acids**, which consist of chains of carbon atoms linked together by chemical bonds. On one end of the carbon chain is a methyl group (a cluster of carbon and hydrogen atoms). On the other end is a carboxyl group (a cluster of carbon, oxygen and hydrogen atoms). The chemical bond between carbon atoms can be either single or double. Single bonds have more hydrogen molecules around them than double bonds. These chemical bonds determine whether a fatty acid is saturated or unsaturated. Fatty acids also come in different lengths: short chain fatty acids have fewer than 6 carbons, while long chain fatty acids have 12 or more carbons.

Fatty acids that are not used up as energy are converted into **triglycerides**. A triglyceride is a molecule formed by attaching three fatty acids onto a glycerol compound that serves as a backbone. Triglycerides are then stored in the body as fat (adipose) tissue.

Saturated fatty acids contain single bonds only. Fats containing saturated fatty acids are called **saturated fats**. Examples of foods high in saturated fats include *ghee,* butter, whole milk, cream, eggs, red meat, and chocolate. An excess intake of saturated fat can raise blood cholesterol.

Monounsaturated fatty acids (MUFA) contain one double bond. Examples of foods high in monounsaturated fat include nuts, olives, and their oils. Increased consumption of **monounsaturated fats** is beneficial in lowering LDL (low density lipoprotein) cholesterol .

Polyunsaturated fatty acids (PUFA) contain more than one double bond. Examples of foods high in **polyunsaturated fats** include vegetable oils, corn, sunflower, and soy.

Essential fatty acids are polyunsaturated fatty acids that the human body needs for metabolic functioning but cannot produce, and therefore has to be acquired from food.

Omega-3 fatty acids e.g. (the alpha linolenic acid) are a class of essential polyunsaturated fatty acids with the double bond in the third carbon position from the methyl group. Foods high in omega-3 fatty acids include salmon, halibut, sardines, trout, herring, walnut, flaxseed oil, and canola oil. Other foods that contain omega-3 fatty acids include shrimp, clams, tuna, catfish, cod, and spinach. Omega-6 fatty acids e.g. (the linoleic acid) are a class of essential polyunsaturated fatty acids with the initial double bond in the sixth carbon position from the methyl group. Examples of foods rich in omega-6 fatty acids include corn, safflower, sunflower, soyabean, and cottonseed oil. Omega-3 and omega-6 fatty acids are also referred to as n-3 and n-6 fatty acids, respectively.

Trans fatty acids have an unusual configuration about their double bond. They (trans fats) are made through hydrogenation (adding hydrogen) to solidify liquid oils. Heating omega-6 oils, such as corn oil, to high temperatures also creates trans fats. Trans fats increase the shelf life of oils and are found in vegetable margarines, commercial pastries, fried foods, cookies, and snack foods. The intake of trans fatty acids increases LDL, and decreases HDL (high density lipoprotein).

Fat in our body

There are three types of fats (lipids) in our body: cholesterol, triglycerides, and phospholipids. All animal fats contain cholesterol. Triglycerides and phospholipids are formed in our body during the digestive process. The fats of a meal are broken down by digestive secretions containing the enzyme lipase with the help of bile salts from the liver. The breakdown products are then absorbed through the intestinal wall and are recombined to form triglycerides and phospholipids. These lipids, in the form of very small droplets (chylomicrons), are transported in blood to points of utilization or storage in the body. If the energy requirement of the body increases, the stored lipids then break down to provide it.

Triglycerides are carried in the blood by very low density lipoproteins (VLDL). Only a small amount of triglycerides is normally found in the blood; mostly it is stored in fat tissue. People with high triglycerides often have high cholesterol levels. Many people with heart disease also have high triglyceride levels. People with diabetes or who are obese are also likely to have high triglycerides. Triglyceride levels of less than 150 mg/dL are normal; levels from 150-199 are borderline high. Levels that are borderline high or high (200 mg/dL to 499 mg/dL) may need treatment in some people. Triglyceride levels of 500 mg/dL or above are very high, and need to be treated definitely.

Sources of fat

Saturated fats: These are the biggest dietary cause of high LDL levels (bad cholesterol). When looking at a food label, pay very close attention to the % of saturated fat and avoid or limit any foods that are high (over 20% saturated fat). Saturated fats are found in animal products such as *ghee*, butter, cheese, whole milk, ice cream, cream, and fatty meats. They are also found in some vegetable oils: coconut, palm, and palm kernel oils (most other vegetable oils contain unsaturated fats and are healthy).

Unsaturated fats: Fats that help to lower blood cholesterol if used in place of saturated fats. However, unsaturated fats have a lot of calories, so you still need to limit them. There are two types: **mono-unsaturated** and **polyunsaturated.** Most (not all) liquid vegetable oils are unsaturated. The exceptions include coconut, palm, and palm kernel oils.

Mono-unsaturated fats (MUFA): Fats that help to lower blood cholesterol if used in place of saturated fats. However, mono-unsaturated fats have a lot of calories, so you still need to limit them. Examples include olive and canola oils.

Polyunsaturated fats (PUFA): Fats that help to lower blood cholesterol if used in place of saturated fats. However, polyunsaturated fats have a lot of calories, so you still need to limit them. Examples include safflower, sunflower, corn, and soybean oils.

Trans fats: These fats form when vegetable oil is heated to very high temperature and also by hydrogenation and can raise LDL levels. They can also lower HDL levels (good cholesterol). Trans-fats are found in fried foods, commercial baked goods (confectionaries, cookies), processed foods, and margarines.

Hydrogenated fats: They refer to oils that have become hardened (such as *vanaspati,* hard butter and margarine). Foods made with hydrogenated oils should be avoided because they contain high levels of trans fatty acids. The terms 'hydrogenated' and 'saturated' are related; an oil becomes saturated when hydrogen is added (i.e., becomes hydrogenated).

Partially hydrogenated fats: These are oils that have become partially hardened. Foods made with partially hydrogenated oils should be avoided because they contain high levels of trans fatty acids.

What are oils

Oils are fats that are liquid at room temperature, like the vegetable oils used in cooking. Oils come from many different plants and from fish. Some common oils are: canola oil, corn oil, cottonseed oil, mustard oil, olive oil, rapeseed oil, safflower oil, sesame oil, soybean oil, sunflower oil. Some oils may be used mainly as flavourings, such as walnut oil and almond oil. A number of foods are naturally high in oils, like: nuts, olives, avocados and some fish.

Most oils are high in healthier fats called monounsaturated (MUFA) or polyunsaturated (PUFA) fats, and low in unhealthy fats called saturated fats. Oils from plant sources (vegetable and nut oils) do not contain any cholesterol. In fact, **no foods from plant sources contain cholesterol.** A few plant oils, however, including coconut oil and palm kernel oil, are high in saturated fats and should be limited in the diet.

Unrefined oils (cold-pressed or filtered) should be used as much as possible. Refining the oil modifies the chemical nature of PUFA, reducing their nutritional value. Vitamin E and lecithin, required for proper utilisation and absorption of fatty acids, also get destroyed in the refining process.

What are solid fats

Most solid fats are high in saturated fats and/or trans fats and have less monounsaturated or polyunsaturated fats. Animal products containing solid fats also contain cholesterol. Trans fats can be found in cakes, cookies, crackers, icings, margarines, and microwave popcorns.

Solid fats are fats that are solid at room temperature, such as butter and vegetable margarine. Solid fats come from many animal foods and can be made from vegetable oils through a process called hydrogenation. Some common solid fats are: *ghee*, butter, *vanaspati*, lard, margarine. Foods high in solid fats include: processed cheese, cream, ice cream, well-marbled cuts of meats, beef, bacon, sausages, poultry, most baked confectionaries (cookies, crackers, doughnuts, pastries, and croissants). In some cases, the fat in the foods may be invisible. Cottage cheese and whole milk are high in solid fat, even though it is not visible.

Reccomendations

Saturated fats, trans fats, and cholesterol tend to raise LDL (bad) cholesterol levels in the blood, which in turn increases the risk for heart disease and stroke. To lower the risks, cut back on foods containing saturated fats, trans fats, and cholesterol. Use oil in your cooking instead of solid fats.

- Choose lean, protein-rich foods like soy, fish, skinless chicken, very lean meat, and fat free or skimmed dairy products.
- Eat foods that are naturally low in fat like whole grains, fruits, and vegetables.
- Limit your consumption of fried foods, processed foods, and commercially prepared sweets and baked goods.
- Limit animal products like *ghee*, butter, egg yolks, cheese, whole milk, cream, ice cream, and fatty meats.
- Look at food labels, especially for the level of saturated fat. Avoid or limit foods high in saturated fat (more than 20% on the label).
- Look on food labels for words like 'hydrogenated' or 'partially hydrogenated,' these foods contain saturated fats and trans-fatty acids and should be avoided.
- Include foods containing omega-3 fatty acids in your daily diet, like cold-water fish (salmon, mackerel), flaxseeds (*alsi*), walnuts, soyabean oil.
- Children under two years of age should NOT be on a fat restricted diet because cholesterol and fatty acids are important nutrients for brain development.

❖ It is recommended that everyone over the age of 20 years should have their blood cholesterol levels (preferably complete lipid profile) checked annually.

Blood cholesterol level or lipid profile

Parameter	*Character*	*Normal levels (mg per cent)*
LDL cholesterol	Bad	<130
VLDL cholesterol	Bad	<28
HDL cholesterol	Good	>55
Total cholesterol		200
Triglycerides	Bad	<130

Cholesterol content (mg per 100gm)

Egg (1 yolk)	260
Chicken without skin	60
Chicken with skin	100
Mutton	65
Liver	300
Brain	2,000
Fish	45
Prawns/shrimps	150
Buffalo milk	16
Cow milk	14
Curd/Yoghurt	16
Cream	40
Cheese	100
Paneer	10

Percentage of fatty acids in fats and oils (gm/100gm)

Name	*Saturated Fat*	*Choles-terol*	*PUFA (P)*	*MUFA (M)*	*Omega 6 FA*	*Omega 3 FA*
Safflower	13	–	60	27	78	–
Sunflower	12	–	60	27	66	–
Groundnut	24	–	26	50	30	–
Mustard	8	–	22	70	18	14.5
Til oil	15	–	43	42	44	0.5
Olive Oil	10	–	8	82	8	0.6
Soyabean	15	–	58	27	50	6.5
Rice bran	22	–	37	41	33	–
Flaxseed	8	–	+	+	13	53
Coconut	90	–	3	7	0.8	–
Butter	50	250	8	23	1.8	–
Margarine	14	–	35	29	–	–
Ghee	65	300	3	32	+	+
Almonds	6	–	17	77	+	–
Cashews	14	–	15	71	+	–
Walnuts	5	–	60	55	+	+

Linolenic acid (omega 3 FA)

2 tablespoons ground flaxseed	3.8 gm
1/4 cup walnuts	2.6 gm
1 cup tofu (soyabean paneer)	0.7 gm
1 cup green leafy vegetables	0.1 gm
Almonds	0.0 gm

Part II

What is Cholesterol

Cholesterol is a harmful alien substance that should be avoided at all costs, is a myth. In fact, nothing could be further from the truth. Cholesterol is an essential component in the body. It is found in all the cells of the body, particularly in the brain and nerve cells. Body cells are continually dying and new ones are being made. Cholesterol is a major building block from which cell walls are made. Cholesterol is also used to make a number of other important substances: hormones (including the sex hormones), bile acids and, in conjunction with sunlight on the skin, vitamin D_3. The body uses large quantities of cholesterol every day and the substance is so important that, with the exception of brain cells, every body cell has the ability to make it.

Our body gets cholesterol from two sources: from the foods we eat and from our liver. Although many foods contain cholesterol, the liver actually produces up to 80% of what the body needs. A compensatory system regulates the amount of cholesterol synthesized by the liver, with the increased dietary intake of cholesterol resulting in the liver's decreased synthesis of the compound.

Cholesterol is insoluble in the blood; it must be attached to certain protein complexes called lipoproteins in order to be transported through the bloodstream. Low-density lipoproteins (LDL) transport cholesterol from its site of synthesis in the liver to the various tissues and body cells, where it is separated from the lipoprotein and is used by the cell. High-density lipoproteins (HDL) transport excess or unused cholesterol from the tissues back to the liver, where it is broken down to bile acids and is then excreted.

LDL and HDL cholesterol

The liver not only manufactures and secretes **LDL cholesterol** into the blood; it also removes LDL cholesterol from the blood. A high number of active LDL receptors on the liver's surface are associated with the rapid removal of LDL cholesterol from the blood and lower blood LDL cholesterol levels. A deficiency of LDL receptors is associated with high LDL cholesterol blood levels. Both heredity and diet have a significant influence on a person's LDL, HDL and total cholesterol levels. Familial hypercholesterolemia (FH) is a common inherited disorder whose victims have a diminished number or nonexistent LDL receptors on the surface of liver cells. People with this disorder also tend to develop atherosclerosis and heart attacks during early adulthood. Diets that are high in saturated fats and cholesterol raise the levels of LDL cholesterol in the blood. (Fats are classified as saturated or unsaturated according to their chemical structure. Saturated fats are derived primarily from meat and dairy products and can raise blood cholesterol levels. Some vegetable oils made from coconut, palm, and cocoa are also high in saturated fats.)

When too much LDL cholesterol circulates in the blood, it can slowly build up in the inner walls of the arteries that feed the heart and brain. Together with other substances it can form plaque, a thick, hard deposit that can clog those arteries. This condition is known as **atherosclerosis.** If a clot forms and blocks a narrowed artery, it can cause a heart attack or stroke. The levels of HDL cholesterol and LDL cholesterol in the blood are measured to evaluate the risk of having a heart attack. LDL cholesterol of less than 100 mg/dL is the optimal level, whereas upto 130 mg/dL is near optimal for most people. **A high LDL level (more than 160 mg/dL) reflects an increased risk of heart disease. That's why LDL cholesterol is often called 'bad' cholesterol.**

Lowering LDL cholesterol is currently the primary focus in preventing atherosclerosis, heart attacks and strokes. The benefits of lowering LDL cholesterol include:

- ❖ Reducing or stopping the formation of new cholesterol plaques on the artery walls;
- ❖ Reducing existing cholesterol plaques on the artery walls;
- ❖ Widening narrowed arteries;
- ❖ Preventing the rupture of cholesterol plaques, which initiates blood clot formation;
- ❖ Decreasing the risk of heart attacks; and
- ❖ Decreasing the risk of strokes. The same measures that retard atherosclerosis in coronary arteries also benefit the carotid and cerebral arteries (arteries that deliver blood to the brain).

About one-third to one-fourth of blood cholesterol is carried by high-density lipoprotein (HDL). **HDL is called the 'good' cholesterol because it protects the arteries from the atherosclerotic process.** HDL cholesterol extracts cholesterol particles from the artery walls and transports them to the liver to be disposed through the bile. It also interferes with the accumulation of LDL cholesterol particles in the artery walls.

The risk of atherosclerosis and heart attacks is strongly related to HDL cholesterol levels. Low levels of HDL cholesterol are linked to a higher risk, whereas high HDL cholesterol levels are associated with a lower risk. (Low HDL cholesterol levels [less than 40 mg/dL] increase the risk for heart disease.)

Very low and very high HDL cholesterol levels have shown to run in families. Like LDL cholesterol, lifestyle factors and other conditions influence HDL cholesterol levels. HDL cholesterol levels are lower in persons who smoke cigarettes, eat a lot of sweets, are overweight and inactive, and in patients with type II diabetes mellitus. HDL cholesterol is higher in people who are lean, exercise regularly, and do not smoke cigarettes. Estrogen increases a person's HDL cholesterol, which explains why women generally have higher HDL levels than men do.

For individuals with low HDL cholesterol levels, a high total or LDL cholesterol blood level further increases the incidence of atherosclerosis and heart attacks. Therefore, the combination of high levels of total and LDL cholesterol with low levels of HDL cholesterol is undesirable whereas the combination of low levels of total and LDL cholesterol and high levels of HDL cholesterol is favourable.

In clinical trials involving lowering LDL cholesterol, scientists also studied the effect of HDL cholesterol on atherosclerosis and heart attack rates. They found that even small increases in HDL cholesterol could reduce the frequency of heart attacks. For each 1 mg/dl increase in HDL cholesterol, there is a 2 to 4% reduction in the risk of coronary heart disease.

The total cholesterol to HDL cholesterol ratio (total chol/HDL) is a number that is helpful in estimating the risk of developing atherosclerosis. The number is obtained by dividing total cholesterol by HDL cholesterol. (High ratios indicate a higher risk of heart attacks, whereas low ratios indicate a lower risk). High total cholesterol and low HDL cholesterol increases the ratio and is undesirable. Conversely, high HDL cholesterol and low total cholesterol lowers the ratio and is desirable. An average ratio would be about 4.5. Ideally, one should strive for ratios of 2 or 3 (less than 4).

Lp(a) cholesterol

Lipoprotein (a) (Lp(a)) is a LDL cholesterol particle that is attached to a special protein called apo(a). A person's level of Lp(a) in the blood is genetically inherited. Elevated levels of Lp(a) (higher than 20 mg/dl to 30 mg/dl) in the blood are linked to a greater likelihood of atherosclerosis and heart attacks in both men and women. The risk is even more significant if the Lp(a) cholesterol elevation is accompanied by high LDL/HDL ratios. Certain diseases are associated with elevated Lp(a) levels. Patients on chronic kidney dialysis and those with nephrotic syndrome (kidney disease that causes leakage of blood proteins into the urine) tend to have high levels of Lp(a).

There are many theories as to how Lp(a) causes atherosclerosis, although exactly how Lp(a) accumulates cholesterol plaques on the artery walls has not been well defined. It seems that the lesions in artery walls contain substances that may interact with Lp(a), leading to the build-up of fatty deposits. Most lipid-lowering medications have a limited effect in lowering Lp(a) cholesterol levels. Estrogen has been shown to lower Lp(a) cholesterol levels by approximately 20% in women with elevated Lp(a) cholesterol. Estrogen can also increase HDL cholesterol levels when given to postmenopausal women.

Factors Affecting Cholesterol Levels

A variety of factors can affect our cholesterol levels. They include:

❖ **Heredity:** Our genes influence how high our LDL cholesterol is by affecting how fast LDL is made and removed from the blood. One specific form of inherited high cholesterol that affects 1 in 500 people is familial hypercholesterolemia, which often leads to early heart disease.

❖ **Diet:** Two main nutrients in the foods make the LDL cholesterol level go up: saturated fat, a type of fat found mostly in foods that come from animals; and cholesterol, which comes only from animal products. Saturated fat raises the LDL-cholesterol level more than anything else in the diet. Reducing the amount of saturated fat and cholesterol in the diet is a very important step in reducing our blood cholesterol levels.

- **Weight:** Excess weight tends to increase the LDL cholesterol level. Weight loss helps to lower not only the LDL, but triglycerides as well; and raises HDL cholesterol levels.

- **Exercise:** Regular exercise can lower LDL cholesterol and raise HDL cholesterol levels. Being physically active for 20-30 minutes daily stabilises the cholesterol levels.

- **Age and Gender:** Before the age of menopause, women usually have total cholesterol levels that are lower than those of men the same age. As women and men get older, their blood cholesterol levels rise until about 60 to 65 years of age. After the age of about 50, women often have higher total cholesterol levels than men of the same age.

- **Alcohol:** Alcohol intake increases HDL cholesterol but does not lower LDL cholesterol. Doctors don't know for certain whether alcohol also reduces the risk of heart disease. Drinking too much alcohol can damage the liver and heart muscle, lead to high blood pressure, and raise triglycerides. Because of the risks, alcoholic beverages should not be used as a way to prevent heart disease.

❖ **Smoking:** Smoking lowers HDL cholesterol levels. This trend can be reversed by quitting smoking.

❖ **Stress:** Long term stress has been shown to raise blood cholesterol levels. One way that stress may do this is by affecting our habits and lifestyle. For example, when some people are under stress, they console themselves by eating fatty foods or junk foods. The saturated fat and cholesterol in these foods contribute to increasing the levels of blood cholesterol.

❖ **Other causes:** Certain medications and medical conditions can cause high cholesterol.

Cholesterol Related Disorders

Lipid molecules, such as triglycerides and cholesterol, circulate in the blood and are bound to carrier protein molecules. In certain hereditary metabolic disorders, known as familial hypercholesterolemias, the levels of triglycerides and cholesterol in the blood are high because the mechanisms that remove them are defective. As a result, triglycerides and cholesterol may be deposited in the skin, tendons, and walls of blood vessels, which can lead to coronary heart disease and early death.

Cholesterol may also be raised secondary to certain diseases; e.g., hypothyroidism, some types of kidney disease, bile duct obstruction, and diabetes mellitus. Finally, it is moderately raised by a diet rich in saturated fat and cholesterol.

Cholelithiasis, or the formation of gallstones in the gallbladder, is the most common disease of the biliary tract. Gallstones are of three types: stones containing primarily calcium bilirubinate (pigment stones); stones containing 25 percent or more of cholesterol; and stones composed of variable mixtures of both bilirubin and cholesterol (mixed gallstones).

Cholesterol and mixed cholesterol-bilirubinate stones occur when the proportion of cholesterol in bile exceeds the capacity of bile acids and lecithin to contain the total amount of cholesterol in micellar colloidal solution. When this critical micellar concentration is surpassed and the solution is saturated, crystalline particles of cholesterol are formed. The resulting gallstones contain large amounts of crystalline cholesterol and smaller quantities of calcium bilirubinate. Cholesterol gallstones occur about twice as frequently in women as they do in men, and at younger ages. Those at increased risk of cholesterol gallstones include persons who are obese, on diets high in caloric content or in cholesterol, diabetics, or taking female sex hormones. Each of these factors favours increased concentration of cholesterol in bile.

In addition, some persons are unable, for genetic reasons, to convert sufficient amounts of cholesterol to bile acids, thus favouring the increased formation of stones. Some illnesses reduce the capacity of the lower small intestine to reabsorb bile acids, leading to deficits of bile acids that cannot be overcome by hepatic synthesis alone. During pregnancy, the ratio of chenodeoxycholic acid to cholic acid in hepatic bile is reduced, thus making bile more prone to produce stones (lithogenic). Decreased flow of bile in the gallbladder, a condition that occurs late in pregnancy, in persons on diets low in fat, and among certain diabetics, also appears to favour the formation of cholesterol stones.

High levels of cholesterol in the bloodstream is an extremely important cause of **atherosclerosis**. In this disorder, cholesterol-carrying lipoproteins in the circulating blood are gradually deposited on the inner linings of arteries over a period of years. As more cholesterol is deposited on the lining, initially tiny lesions enlarge and thicken to form plaques, narrowing the vessel channel and interfering with the flow of blood through it. The formation of fatty deposits may also be accompanied by scar tissue and calcification, which make the vessel walls less elastic, one consequence being an increase in blood pressure. Eventually an arterial channel may be completely blocked by thick plaques, or a blood clot (thrombus) may form at the site of a plaque and obstruct the channel.

When atherosclerosis affects the coronary arteries, which bring oxygen-rich blood to the heart muscle, it can decrease the supply of blood to the heart muscle and result in the pain of angina pectoris, better known as **heart attack**. The complete occlusion of one or more coronary arteries can cause the death of a section of the heart muscle (myocardial infarction).

Atherosclerosis affecting the cerebral blood vessels may interfere with blood flow to the brain and result in a **stroke**, a loss of consciousness followed by some degree of paralysis.

Atherosclerosis affecting the peripheral arteries may reduce blood flow to the legs and cause intermittent lameness and ulceration. There is also an increased possibility of infection in the feet and legs.

Cholesterol-lowering Prescription

High and very high risk people: For high-risk patients, the overall goal remains an LDL level of less than 100 mg/dL. But for very high-risk patients whose LDL levels are already below 100 mg/dL, there is also an option to use drug therapy to go below 70 mg/dL goal. High-risk people are those who have coronary heart disease or disease of the blood vessels of the brain or extremities, or diabetes, or multiple (2 or more) risk factors (e.g., smoking, hypertension). Very high-risk people are those who have cardiovascular disease together with either multiple risk factors (especially diabetes), or severe and poorly controlled risk factors (such as continued smoking), or metabolic syndrome (a combination of risk factors associated with obesity including high triglycerides and low HDL). Patients hospitalized for acute coronary syndromes such as heart attack are also at very high risk.

Moderately high-risk people: For moderately high-risk patients, the goal remains an LDL level under 130 mg/dL, but there is a therapeutic option to set a lower LDL goal of under 100 mg/dL and to use drug therapy at LDL levels of 100 – 129 mg/dL to reach this lower goal. Moderately high-risk patients are those who have multiple (2 or more) risk factors for coronary heart disease. For high-risk or moderately high-risk patients, it is advised to take the cholesterol-lowering drugs and follow the diet and lifestyle regime as suggested in this book.

Lower/moderate risk people: Those people with only one risk factor for coronary heart disease are at a low/moderate risk. For them the cholesterol-busting diet and lifestyle regime, as recommended in this book is sufficient. Lifestyle changes (good nutrition, physical activity, and weight control) continue to be very important in cholesterol management, as they also have the potential to reduce cardiovascular risks through several mechanisms beyond the lowering of LDL cholesterol.

Medications to lower cholesterol

Medications are prescribed when lifestyle changes cannot reduce the LDL cholesterol to desired levels. Various medications are used to lower blood cholesterol levels. They may be prescribed individually or in combination with other drugs. Some of the common types of cholesterol-lowering drugs include statins, resins, nicotinic acid (niacin), gemfibrozil and clofibrate.

Statins: Statin drugs are very effective for lowering LDL cholesterol levels and have few immediate short-term side effects. They interrupt the formation of cholesterol from the circulating blood. Commonly prescribed statins include:

- ❖ Atorvastatin (Lipitor)
- ❖ Fluvastatin (Lescol)
- ❖ Lovastatin (Mevacor)
- ❖ Pravastatin (Pravachol)
- ❖ Rosuvastatin Calcium (Crestor)
- ❖ Simvastatin (Zocor)

Resins: Resins are also called bile-acid binding drugs. They work in the intestines by promoting increased disposal of cholesterol. There are three kinds of medications in this class: Cholestyramine

(Questran, Prevalite, Lo-Cholest); Colestipol (Colestid); Colesevelam (WelChol)

Nicotinic acid: This drug works in the liver by affecting the production of blood fats. It is used to lower triglycerides and LDL cholesterol, and raise HDL cholesterol.

Gemfibrozil (lopid): This drug raises HDL cholesterol levels.

Clofibrate (atromid-S): This drug raises the HDL cholesterol levels and lowers triglyceride levels.

All the above medications have to be prescribed by your physician because of their serious potential side-effects.

Alternate therapies

Homeopathy: Aconite, Arg nit, Arsenicum, Gelsemium, Phosphorus are recommended.

Aromatherapy: Amber (essential oil) is recommended.

Herbal remedies: Ashwagandha, Astragalus, Boneset, Red Root, Siberian Ginseng are recommended.

One thing must be mentioned here about alternate therapies, that it should not be taken without the guidance of the master of the field. In all of them, one person's medicine could be the other's poison.

Diet prescription to lower cholesterol

Dietary change is the first line of intervention for patients with lipid disorders. Saturated fats should be replaced by mono and polyunsaturated fatty acids. By lowering LDL cholesterol, a person is able to significantly reduce the risk of heart disease and accompanying health complications. Current dietary advice focuses on the restriction of saturated fatty acids and cholesterol intake, combined with exercise and ideal body weight. And lowering one's cholesterol through diet usually doesn't require sticking to a very strict diet - simple dietary changes can lower cholesterol just as effectively.

To begin with, simply increasing the intake of fresh fruits and vegetables, whole cooked grains, legumes, nuts and seeds, and eating less meat, cheese, restaurant food and packaged foods, limiting the fat intake exclusively (or nearly so) to limited amounts of pure unrefined oil, and ensuring that you exercise daily for at least 30 minutes will go a long way towards lowering your blood cholesterol.

The table here outlines important dietary elements and how they affect the total cholesterol level:

Effect of different foods on our cholesterol level

Dietary element	*Found in which foods*	*Effect on our cholesterol level*
Alcohol *	Red wine, White wine	Moderate consumption (0–1 glasses per day for a woman; 1–2 per day for men) may improve HDL.
	Hard liquor	More than 2 drinks (30ml each) per day may raise triglyceride levels significantly in overweight people or those with elevated triglyceride levels. Heavy drinking significantly increases risk of heart and liver damage, addiction, and other serious health problems.
Dietary cholesterol	Egg yolks, Red meat (especially organ meats), Dairy products (other than skimmed milk), Hydrogenated cooking mediums	Total blood cholesterol is raised.
Dietary fibre	Beans, Legumes, Whole grains, Soy, Nuts, Citrus fruits, Vegetables	Proven to reduce total cholesterol and LDL.

* Doctors do not generally recommend drinking alcohol to raise the HDL cholesterol level, and one should not do so without first consulting the doctor.

Role of carbohydrates

There are two main sources of dietary carbohydrates: Simple sugars, such as sucrose (the sugar added to sweets and desserts), fructose (the sugar contained in fruit), and lactose (milk sugar); and complex carbohydrates, which come from vegetables and grains.

Most of our carbohydrate calories should come from complex carbohydrates. Foods with complex carbohydrates, as opposed to refined sugars, contain vitamins, minerals, and fibre.

Common Misconceptions About Cholesterol

1. Using margarine instead of butter will help lower cholesterol.

Both margarine and butter are high in fat, so both are to be used in moderation. From a dietary perspective, the major factor affecting blood cholesterol is how much saturated fat is in the food. Reducing the intake of saturated fat is the key to helping control cholesterol.

2. Thin people do not have to worry about high cholesterol.

Overweight people are more likely to have high cholesterol from eating too many fatty foods, but thin people should also have their cholesterol checked regularly. Often people who don't gain weight easily are less aware of how much saturated fat they eat. Nobody can "eat anything they want" and stay heart healthy. Cholesterol levels should be checked regularly regardless of our weight, exercise habits and diet. Highly stressed thin people are known to have high cholesterol levels and are more prone to heart attacks and strokes.

3. My doctor hasn't said anything about my cholesterol, so I don't have to worry.

Unfortunately, not all physicians are as proactive about healthy lifestyles as they should be. Our health is our responsibility. We should make sure that we have our cholesterol levels checked and learn how to interpret all the numbers, including HDL cholesterol, LDL cholesterol and triglyceride levels. If we are in a high or borderline-high range, we may be able to control the levels by eating a diet lower in saturated fat and cholesterol, getting 20 minutes of physical activity daily and quitting smoking. If lifestyle changes alone don't work, our physician may prescribe a cholesterol-lowering medication.

4. Since I am on medication for my high cholesterol, I may eat what I want.

Unless the cholesterol is dangerously high, it's best to try to reduce it by changing the diet. Drug therapy is usually prescribed for those who, despite adequate dietary changes, regular physical activity and weight loss, still have elevated levels of cholesterol. Modern medications have come a long way in helping to control blood cholesterol levels, but making lifestyle changes along with taking medication is the best way to help prevent heart disease. Reducing the amount of saturated fat and cholesterol in the diet and getting 30–60 minutes of exercise on most or all days of the week is recommended, even on cholesterol-lowering medication. It's also very important to take the medication exactly as the doctor has instructed so it can work most efficiently. "I may eat what I want" should not be encouraged as it will slow down the effect of the medication.

5. Women do not have to worry. High cholesterol is a man's problem.

Pre-menopausal women are usually protected from high levels of LDL cholesterol, because the female hormone oestrogen tends to raise HDL cholesterol levels. Post-menopausal women may find that even a heart-healthy diet and regular exercise aren't enough to keep their cholesterol from rising. If you're approaching menopause, it's especially important to have your cholesterol checked and talk with your doctor about your options.

6. Cholesterol need not be checked until one reaches middle age.

It's a good idea to start having our cholesterol checked at an early age. Even children, especially those in families with a history of heart disease, can have high cholesterol levels. And evidence exists that these children are at greater risk for developing heart disease as adults. Lack of exercise, poor dietary habits and genetics can all affect a child's cholesterol levels. One is never too young to develop a heart-healthy lifestyle by eating foods low in saturated fats, getting 30 minutes of physical activity on most days, and avoiding tobacco products.

PART III

Natural Cholesterol Busters

After having understood how to lower our intake of cholesterol, it is fairly simple to monitor our diet. The task now at hand is to remove the extra cholesterol stored in our bodies. One method already discussed is the prescription of medicines. Here we will see how nature has been so kind to provide cholesterol-busters to us. These natural compounds are freely available in foods all around us. It is true that if the problem comes from food then its solution also lies in food.

1. Alpha-linolenic acid (major component of the omega-3 fatty acids)

Omega-3 fatty acids are a part of PUFA (polyunsaturated fatty acids) family. Since the body can not make them, these essential fatty acids have to be sourced from the diet. Omega-3 fatty acids have been shown to play a part in keeping cholesterol and triglyceride levels low, stabilizing irregular heart beat (arrhythmia), and reducing blood pressure. They are the main components of nerve cells and cell membranes throughout the body. They transport oxygen from red blood cells to the body's tissues. They also regulate the release of inflammatory chemicals from cells, controlling inflammation of the arteries. The dietary sources of omega-3s are: spinach, mustard greens, wheat germ, walnuts, flaxseeds, pumpkin seeds, canola, kidney beans, soyabeans, salmon, tuna, herring and sardines.

Key omega-3 fatty acids include Eicosapentaenoic acid (EPA) and Docosahexanoic acid (DHA), both found primarily in oily cold-water fish such as tuna, salmon, and mackerel. Aside from fresh seaweed or spirulina, plant foods rarely contain EPA or DHA. However, a third omega-3, called Alpha-linolenic acid (ALA), is found primarily in flaxseed oil and walnuts. Researchers now believe that Alpha-linolenic acid (ALA) is particularly beneficial for protecting against heart and vessel disease, and for lowering cholesterol and triglyceride levels. It acts as a precursor to prostaglandins, which are hormone-like chemicals that affect everything from heart rate and blood clotting to the constriction and dilatation of blood vessels. It is a natural blood thinner, reducing the 'stickiness' of blood cells (called platelet aggregation). Excellent sources of ALA are flaxseeds, walnuts, canola and soyabean oil.

One to two tablespoons of ground flaxseeds daily in the diet is recommended, mixed with cereal, salad or soups, to break down the cholesterol deposits in the blood vessels. Flaxseed oil, walnuts and walnut oil are also suggested, to be consumed uncooked. For non-vegetarians, increasing the fish intake (to 2-3 times a week) in the diet is advised.

Omega-3s not only keep the body free from heart disease, but also stave off problems like arthritis, pre-menstrual syndrome, asthma, depression, psoriasis and certain types of cancer.

2. Antioxidants

Antioxidants are substances in food that stop it from getting oxidised. This means that they stop fats from turning rancid. Antioxidants are also produced naturally in the body. Certain vitamins are called 'antioxidant nutrients,' as they protect the heart by reducing the production of harmful chemicals in the blood such as the free radicals. These are unstable chemicals generated naturally in the body. Scientists believe that free radicals speed up the process of the hardening of the arteries. There is evidence that cholesterol gets oxidised before it develops or settles within the artery walls, and antioxidants help prevent this process.

Beta-carotene is the best known of the carotenoids, which are the red, orange, and yellow pigments giving colour to fruits and vegetables. The body converts beta-carotene into vitamin A. Also it is a potent immune-system booster and a powerful antioxidant. Carotenoids and cholesterol share a common metabolic pathway, and a high intake of carotenoids is found to block cholesterol synthesis.

Vitamin E is actually an umbrella term for a group of compounds called tocopherols and tocotrienols. Wheat germ, almonds, peanuts, vegetable oils (safflower, corn, and soyabean), green leafy vegetables, and walnuts are just a few prime sources of this powerful antioxidant. Taken together, the combination of beta-carotene and vitamin E is known to lower cholesterol and prevent its oxidation as well.

Flavonoids are natural chemicals found abundantly in plants. They are present in fruit and vegetables especially in apples and onions. One can also get them in red wine, beer, ale, stout and tea. Chemically they are known as polyphenols. Research indicates that flavonoids have potent antioxidant properties and this may reduce oxidation of low-density lipoproteins, the harmful type of cholesterol. Also, some evidence suggests that flavonoids have some effect on blood platelets making them less sticky, so possibly reducing the risk of a blood clot.

Pterostilbene is an antioxidant, similar to **Resveratrol**, which is found in grapes. It reduces the levels of bad cholesterol, and other blood fats by stimulating a receptor protein in liver cells. Resveratrol's antioxidant properties also help in reducing the oxidation of LDL cholesterol.

3. Fibre

Dietary fibre is normally found in unprocessed plant foods. It is a low energy nutrient not digested completely by the human body and thereby helping in the excretion of toxic wastes from the system.

Most foods contain a mixture of soluble and insoluble fibre, which together make up the dietary fibre family. Compounds that dissolve or swell when put into water are called **soluble** fibres and include pectin, gums and mucilage. These compounds are found inside and around plant cells and exist as gum arabic, guar gum, locust bean gum, and pectin. Soluble fibre present in vegetables, lentils, fruits, nuts, beans, oats and barley, has a cholesterol lowering effect. It has been found to bind itself to the cholesterol molecules in the intestines and thus inhibiting its absorption by the blood stream. Soluble fibre also inhibits the bile recycling in the intestinal tract. Bile, which is formed from cholesterol, is pulled into the faeces for elimination, rather than eventually accumulating in the blood.

Insoluble fibre is considered a 'noncarbohydrate carbohydrate' since the components that make up insoluble fibre are lignin, cellulose, and hemicellulose. All of these compounds form the structural parts of plants and do not readily dissolve in water and are not metabolised by intestinal bacteria. Insoluble fibres found in plants like leafy vegetables, peas, beans absorb the cholesterol from the digested food mixture in the intestine. Since the body in this manner excretes the excess cholesterol, the blood cholesterol levels are lowered.

Dietary Fibre Content of Some Common Indian Foods

Food	*Dietary Fibre (g/100 g)*
Cereals and millets	
Rice	7.6
Wheat	17.6
Sorghum	14.3
Bajra	20.3
Ragi	18.6
Pulses and legumes	
Green gram dal	13.5
Black gram dal	14.3
Red gram dal	14.1
Bengal gram dal	13.6
Nuts and oilseeds	
Groundnut	6.1
Coconut dry (copra)	8.9
Roots and tubers	
Sweet potato	7.3
Potato	4.0
Yam	5.3
Fruits	
Banana	2.5
Mango	2.3
Vegetables	
Amaranth	3.4
Palak	5.0
Brinjal	2.0
Ridge gourd	5.7
Snake gourd	1.8
Bottle gourd	2.8
Yellow pumpkin	0.5

Source: B.S. Narasinga Rao, Nutrition Foundation of India Bulletin, 9: (4) 1988.

4. Guggulsterone

The resin of the Commiphora mukul tree has been used in Ayurvedic medicine for more than 2000 years to treat a variety of ailments. Most studies have shown that this resin or gum, termed *guggul*, can decrease elevated lipid levels. Guggulsterone has been identified as the active agent in this resin. Since the 1980s, an extract of the resin, dubbed guggulipid, is being marketed as a cholesterol lowering agent. Additional studies show *guggul* to lower blood pressure and having anti inflammatory activity as well.

5. Niacin

Also known as vitamin B_3 or nicotinic acid, niacin has earned a reputation (in a supplement form) as a natural cholesterol-lowering agent that often rivals prescription drugs in mild to moderate cases. A dose of 2 to 3 grams per day (an average diet would contain 15-30 mg of niacin per day) added to the prescribed statin drugs is a common practice. It may also help to prevent or treat a number of other disorders, from arthritis and depression to diabetes. Unlike most prescription cholesterol-lowering medications, which simply lower levels of LDL cholesterol and triglycerides, niacin is most effective in increasing HDL cholesterol while lowering LDL cholesterol, Lp(a) cholesterol, and triglyceride levels. Niacin is most suited for individuals whose only problem is low HDL cholesterol, as used alone it can raise HDL cholesterol levels by 30% or more. As a result, this vitamin proves to be more potent than conventional medicines in ultimately reducing the risk for a heart attack.

6. Phytosterols

Studies have shown that the use of phytosterols is a very effective way for individuals to lower their LDL cholesterol levels. Plant sterols and plant stanols are collectively known as phytosterols. Plant sterols are plant compounds with chemical structures similar to that of cholesterol. Especially high sterol levels are found in rice bran, wheat germ, corn oil, rye and soyabeans. In a more concentrated form, these substances are called plant stanols.

Structurally these compounds are chemically similar to cholesterol. However, unlike cholesterol derived from animal sources, which gets absorbed easily and raises the body's own cholesterol levels, phytosterols are difficult to absorb. Interestingly, phytosterols so closely resemble cholesterol that they can actually block food-based cholesterol from being absorbed into the bloodstream. The result is that both phytosterols and dietary cholesterol end up being excreted by the body.

Because of their ability to block dietary cholesterol absorption, phytosterols help lower the cholesterol levels. And by lowering total and LDL cholesterol levels, plant sterols and stanols reduce the risk of heart disease. Studies have shown that daily intake of phytosterols can lower cholesterol levels by an average of 10% to 14%.

7. Policosanol

Policosanol is a mixture of waxy substances manufactured from sugarcane or beeswax. It appears to slow down cholesterol synthesis in the liver and also to increase liver reabsorption of LDL (bad) cholesterol. It is approved as a treatment for high cholesterol in many countries. Policosanol also seems to have mild anti-platelet activity which helps in thinning the blood.

Cholesterol Busting Foods

Research has shown how the various cholesterol-busting nutrients of the foods are effective in combating heart disease; it is up to us now to take nature's help in looking after ourselves. From the list below of the cholesterol-busting foods, we should incorporate as many as possible in our daily diet. It is not a difficult task as most of these foods are available most of the time.

Artichoke

Artichokes are high in cynarine, a chemical that stimulates the production of bile, which helps the digestion of fats. This makes it the perfect starter for any rich meal. Good sources of potassium, artichokes help to lower cholesterol. They can be eaten as any other fruit, as salad or mid-morning snack.

Apple

Apples contain fibre, the insoluble one works like bran, latching on to LDL cholesterol in the digestive tract and removing it from the body. Soluble fibre pectin reduces the amount of LDL cholesterol produced in the liver. Eating 2 large apples a day can reduce the cholesterol levels by up to 16 per cent. Apples also contain malic acid, which helps to digest rich fatty foods. Apples can be eaten in any form at any time of the day but stewed apple for breakfast is recommended.

Avocado

Avocados are packed with nutrients. Rich in vitamin A, vitamin E and potassium, they are useful sources of vitamin B6 and mono-unsaturated fatty acids. High in glutathione, an antioxidant that helps to neutralize fat in other foods, they hence help in lowering the total dietary cholesterol. They can be eaten as any other fruit, as salad or mid-morning snack.

Banana

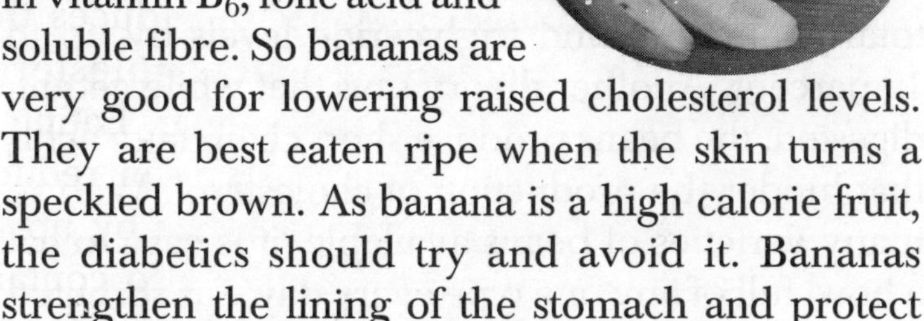

Bananas are highly nutritious for they are very high in potassium and rich in vitamin B_6, folic acid and soluble fibre. So bananas are very good for lowering raised cholesterol levels. They are best eaten ripe when the skin turns a speckled brown. As banana is a high calorie fruit, the diabetics should try and avoid it. Bananas strengthen the lining of the stomach and protect it from excess acidity and ulcers.

Beans

All kinds of beans (including Bengal gram) are rich in the best sort of fibre - soluble fibre - that helps to eliminate cholesterol from the body. They are a good source of folic acid, potassium, copper, phosphorous and manganese. As a high-potassium, low-sodium food they help reduce blood pressure. Not only are they low in fat, but also when combined with grains, beans supply high quality protein that provides a healthy alternative to meat or other animal protein. Beans also contain lecithin, a nutrient that helps dissolve cholesterol. One study showed that a cup and a half of dried lentils or kidney beans a day, about the amount in a bowl of bean soup, could lower total cholesterol and triglyceride levels by up to 19 percent. Another theory says that while getting digested, the beans produce short chain fatty acids that hinder the production of cholesterol. With so many varieties of beans available, it is easy to eat a bowl full of any one type every day – as sprouted salad, boiled bean *chaat*, or simply as curry or *dal*.

Berries

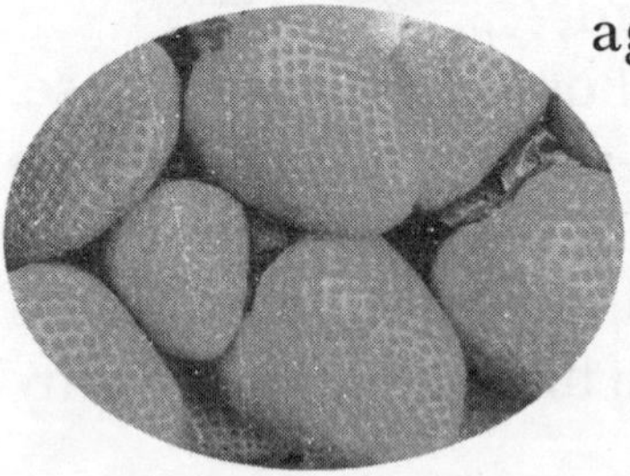

All kinds of berries have cholesterol-busting properties. **Blackberries** are rich in vitamin C and are excellent source of vitamin E, which is beneficial for the heart and circulatory problems. In addition they contain the soluble fibre pectin, which helps to eliminate cholesterol, and protects against environmental toxins. All berries are a good source of potassium as well. **Blueberries** have an antioxidant pterostilbene, which reduces LDL and triglycerides by stimulating the protein receptors of the liver cells. **Raspberries'** phytochemical content includes beta-carotene, ellagic acid, catechins, and monoterpenes (which also inhibit cholesterol production). **Strawberries** contain modest amounts of iron as well. All kinds of berries are perhaps one of the healthiest fruits you can eat. Berries can be eaten fresh as fruit, or raw as pickled in oil (especially *amla, karonda* and *tainti*).

Brinjal (eggplant)

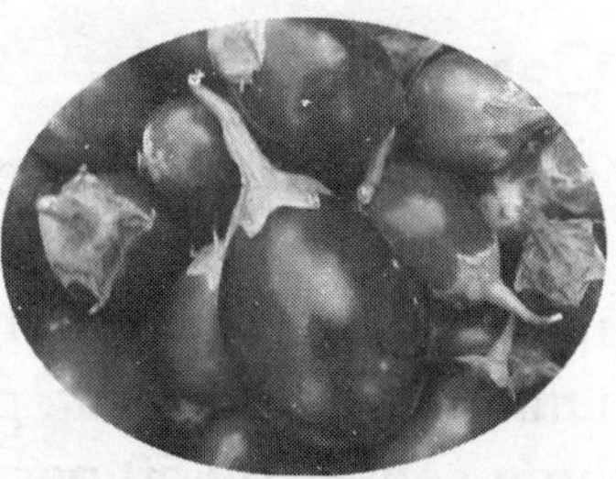

In addition to featuring a host of vitamins and minerals, eggplant also contains important phytonutrients, which have antioxidant activity. They include phenolic compounds, such as caffeic acid and chlorogenic acid, and flavonoids, such as nasunin. Nasunin is a potent antioxidant and free radical scavenger. Eating brinjal as normal vegetable or *bhurta* is quite easily done, as are the *pakoras,* but the best way to eat it is by simply sautéing it lightly in oil, with minimal salt and turmeric powder and eating it with yoghurt.

Broccoli

Like garlic, broccoli is one of today's miracle foods. A member of the brassica family, broccoli is high in cholesterol-busting antioxidant vitamins beta-carotene, vitamin C, vitamin E and rich in folic acid. It also contains iron and potassium. Though eaten as any other cooked vegetable, broccoli is best as steamed in salads.

Carrot

The beta-carotene present in carrots lowers the cholesterol. A couple of carrots a day can reduce the cholesterol levels by up to 10 per cent, heart attack by 22 per cent, paralysis by 40 per cent and lung cancer by 50 per cent. Carrots are also high in the fibre pectin. Carrot juice - raw or fermented, pickled carrots, carrot *halwa* or as vegetable preparations, are the most commonly used methods of consuming carrots. All are good but the best remains eating it raw as salad.

Citrus fruits

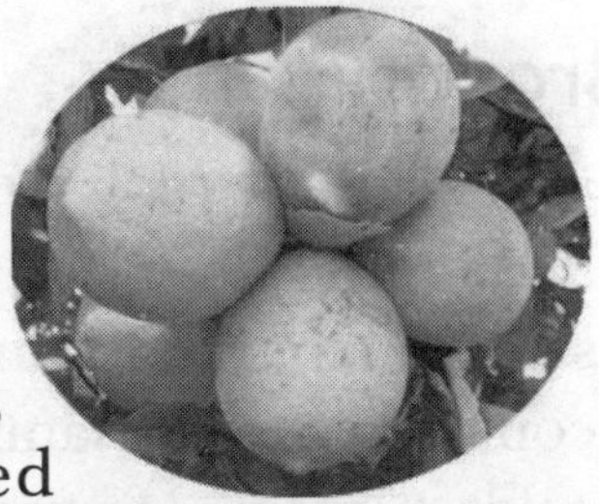

Pectin (more in the rind and core of all the citrus fruits) reduces the cholesterol dramatically. Compounds, called polymethoxylated flavones (PMFs), tangeretin and nobiletin, found in the peels of **tangerines** and **oranges** have the most potent cholesterol-lowering effect. A Dutch study found that citrus fruit, probably because of its supply of the B vitamin folic acid, lowers blood levels of homo-cysteine, a substance that may increase the risk of heart disease. **Grapefruit** is high in vitamin C, potassium, several carotenoids including beta-carotene. The white pith contains pectin and bioflavonoids which makes grapefruit the best antioxidant citrus fruit. The easiest way to use the citrus benefits is to drink a glass of grapefruit juice for breakfast, and use lime in salads generously.

Fish

Fish is extremely nutritious and a good source of protein. White fish such as haddock and cod are also low in fat and contain high levels of vitamin B12, their livers are rich in oils which contain

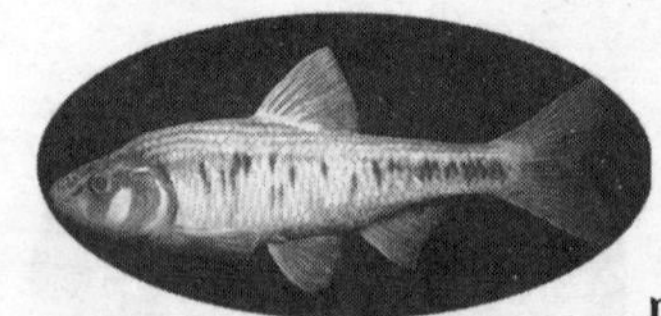

vitamins A and D, plus omega-3 fatty acids. Oily fish, which includes tuna, nackerel, sardines and salmon, are higher in calories than white fish, but contain more unsaturated fats and omega-3 fatty acids. Omega-3 fatty acids are extremely beneficial for the heart. Research has shown that fish oil supplementation is highly effective in reducing triglyceride levels and lowering the triglyceride/HDL ratio. It has been found that taking 8 fish oil capsules daily (providing 2.4 grams of Eicosapentaenoic acid and 1.6 grams of Docosahexaenoic acid) reduced triglyceride levels by about 26% and triglyceride/HDL ratio by 28% in women. Another study found an average reduction of 38% in triglyceride levels and an increase of HDL levels of 24% in both men and women consuming fish on a daily basis. The triglyceride-reducing effect is unique to long-chain omega-3 acids found in fish oils. It is recommended to have fish at least two to three times in a week.

Flaxseed (Linseed)

Flaxseed is a rich source of polyunsaturated fats and mono-unsaturated fats. It contains nearly two and a half times as much omega-3 as omega-6. It also contains vitamins, minerals, protein, and lignan (helps in preventing certain types of cancers). Flaxseed contains about 14 grams of omega-3 per 100gm, which makes it a premium vegetarian food source of omega-3. Because of its high essential fatty acid content, flaxseed lowers blood cholesterol and triglyceride levels. It also reduces inflammation (in arthritis) and promotes skin health. Adding 2 tablespoons of flaxseeds (roasted and ground if desired) to your daily diet can fulfill your daily requirement of essential fatty acids, plus provide calcium, magnesium and zinc. Flaxseed oil is best used raw as in salad dressings, though it can also be used blended together with soyabean oil, pumpkin seed oil or sesame oil.

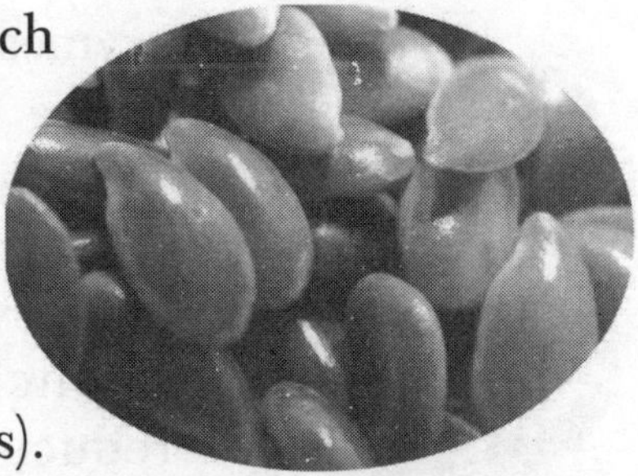

Garlic

Garlic appears to be a miracle food. It contains the compound allicin which has anti-bacterial effects and helps reduce unhealthy fats and cholesterol. Allicin blocks the action of bacterial enzymes by reacting with thiols. Since thiols are also crucial components of some enzymes that participate in the synthesis of cholesterol, hence the cholesterol reducing property of garlic. Garlic also contains antioxidants that reduce blood clotting as well. Garlic is best eaten raw, roasted or pickled in limejuice. If frying garlic, do *not* allow it to get brown. Garlic prevents the growth of tumours.

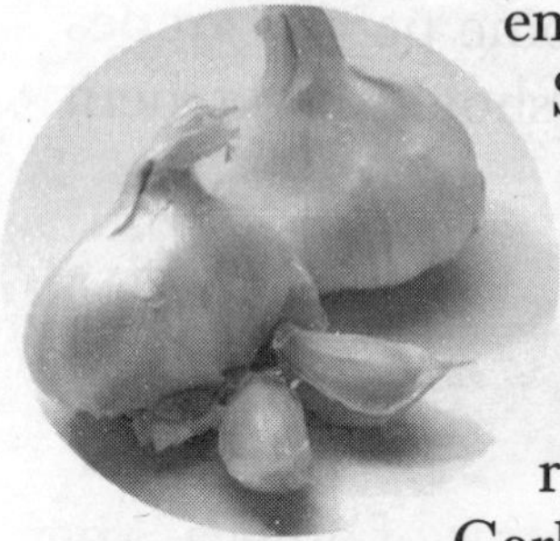

Grapes

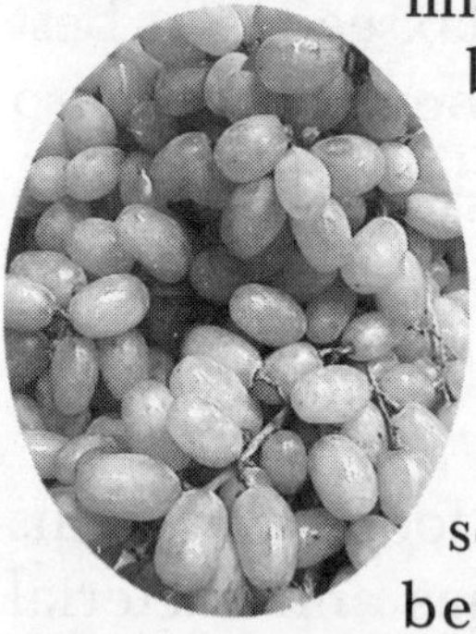

Grapes are rich in anthocyanins, flavones, geraniol, linalol, nerol and tannins. Experts believe these compounds to have antioxidant activity. In addition, red grapes contain resveratrol, which is believed to help reduce cholesterol and protect the heart. Grapes also contain some potassium and are also beneficial for cleansing and detoxifying the system. Eating grapes as mid-morning snack is recommended, but care should be taken not to overeat as in some people grapes may cause diarrhoea. Diabetics should avoid them as grapes are very high in calories.

Green tea

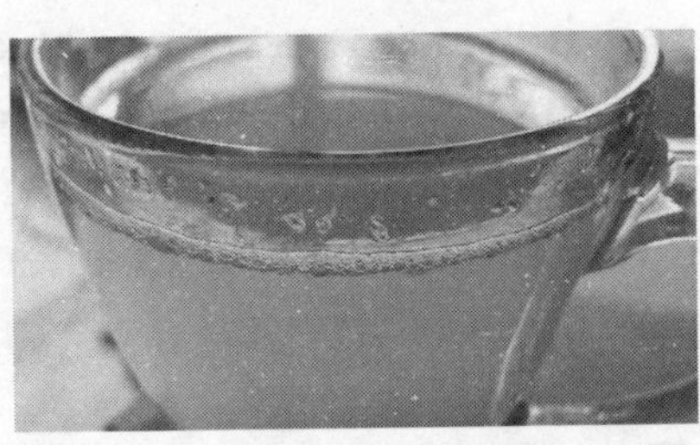

There is research indicating that drinking green tea lowers total cholesterol levels, as well as improve the ratio of good (HDL) cholesterol to bad (LDL) cholesterol. The secret of green tea lies in the fact that it is rich in catechin polyphenols, particularly epigallocatechin gallate (EGCG). EGCG is a powerful antioxidant; besides inhibiting the growth of cancer cells, it has also been effective in lowering LDL cholesterol levels, and inhibiting the abnormal formation of blood clots. Green, oolong (a kind of darkcoloured partly fermented China tea), and black teas come from the leaves of the Camellia sinensis plant. What sets green tea apart is the way it is processed. Green tea leaves are steamed, which prevents the EGCG compound from being oxidised. By contrast, black and oolong tea leaves are made from fermented leaves, which results in the EGCG being converted into other compounds that are not nearly as effective in preventing and fighting various diseases. According to the researchers, epicatechins present in jasmine tea block cholesterol absorption and increase excretion of cholesterol-containing bile salts and fatty acids. The chemicals also speed the breakdown of triglycerides to fatty acids so they can be burned as energy. Drinking a cup of green tea is advised after lunch and dinner.

Guava

Guavas are extremely rich in vitamin C and are useful sources of calcium, nicotinic acid, phosphorous, and soluble fibre. They are very good for the immune system and are beneficial in reducing cholesterol and protecting the heart. Guavas are best eaten fresh.

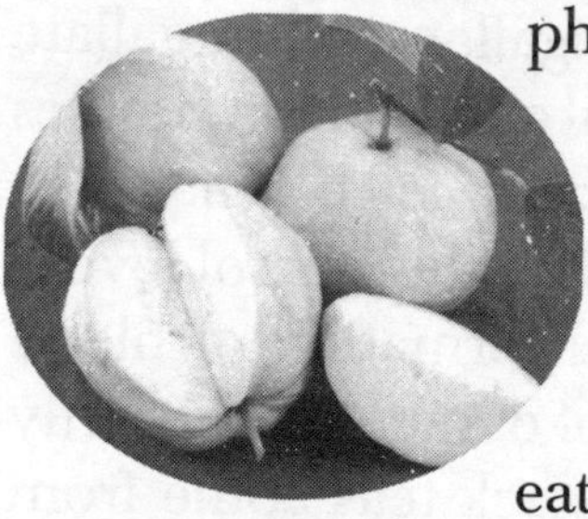

Mushroom

Mushrooms provide a wealth of protein, fibre, B vitamins, and vitamin C, as well as calcium and other minerals. Research has showed the benefits of **shiitake** mushroom in lowering cholesterol. In

Japan, they have identified a specific amino acid in shiitake that helps speed up the processing of cholesterol in the liver. In a study reported in 1997, 40 elderly individuals and 420 young women consumed nine grams of dried shiitake or the equivalent amount of fresh shiitake (90g) every day for 7 days. After a week, total cholesterol levels had dropped 7 to 15% in the older group, and 6 to 12% in the young women. Mushrooms can be consumed raw in salads or cooked in soups, vegetables and curries.

Mustard and Fenugreek

Mustard and fenugreek belong to the same family and are consumed in food as seeds, leaves and oil. High in fibre (in leaves) and alkaloids (in seeds), they are very effective in reducing the cholesterol, triglyceride and sugar levels in the blood. Mustard oil has been found equally effective as corn oil and sunflower oil in reducing plasma total and

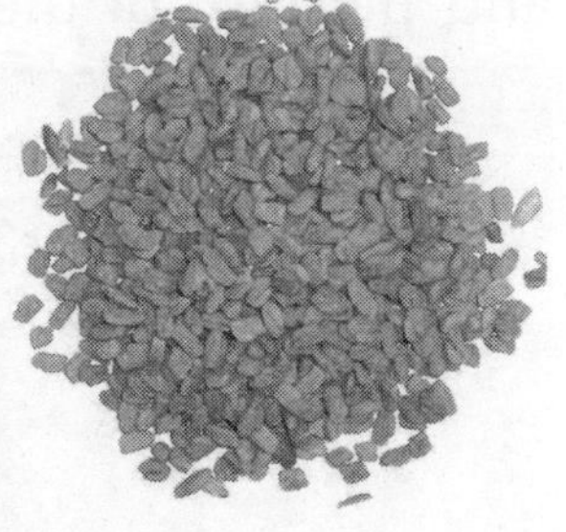

LDL Cholesterol levels. Mustard oil has 30 per cent protein, calcium, phytins, phenolics and natural antioxidants. It contains high amount of mono-unsaturated fatty acids and a good ratio of polyunsaturated fatty acids, which is good for heart. Glucosinolate, the pungent principle in mustard oil, has anti bacterial, anti fungal and anti-carcinogenic properties, which account for many medicinal utilities of the oil. Apart from being consumed as a cooking medium and in pickles, mustard oil can be used raw as a salad dressing with fruits like apples and pears.

Nuts

All nuts are an excellent source of protein and fibre and minerals including selenium, zinc and magnesium, and contain useful amounts of phosphorous, copper and iron. **Almonds** have the highest protein content as compared to other nuts, and because of their high monounsaturated fat

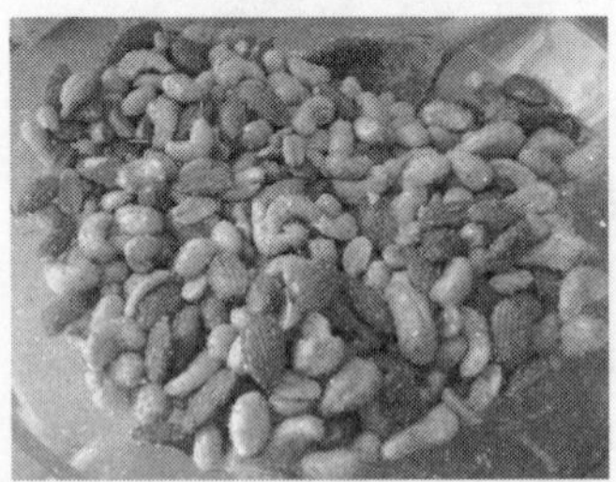

content, significantly reduce total and LDL cholesterol levels. Almonds also contain a high degree of oleic acid, which is believed to be the ingredient in olive oil that protects against heart disease. **Brazil nuts** have about 2,500 times as much selenium as any other nut. Selenium is a powerful antioxidant, which has been proven to protect against heart disease. **Cashew nuts** are also rich in mono-unsaturated fat that helps protect the heart. Cashew nuts are also a good source of potassium, B vitamins and folate. **Walnuts** are rich in omega-3 fatty acids that significantly reduce the LDL and are also a source of sterols and some flavonoids. Walnuts are low in saturated fat and high in both polyunsaturated and mono-unsaturated fat. Walnuts are a good source of protein, vitamin B_1, B_6, folate and vitamin E. Green and unripe walnuts are rich in vitamin C. Research has found that eating regular amounts of walnuts or almonds reduces bad cholesterol (LDL) in the blood. The best time to eat nuts is breakfast, or as a mid-day snack.

Olive

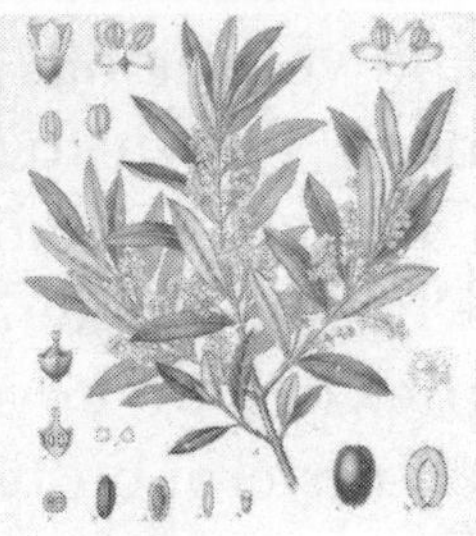

Olive oil is a mono-unsaturated fat. Mono-unsaturated fats reduce the capacity of LDL cholesterol to oxidise, which may explain the protective properties of olive oil. However, extra virgin olive oil also contains around 40 antioxidant phytochemicals. Antioxidants are associated with reduced oxidation of LDL cholesterol. Olive oil is by far the best cholesterol-busting cooking medium, but can also be used as salad dressing.

Onion

The common onion possesses the medicinal properties that are very similar to those of garlic. It has antimicrobial qualities, reduces blood pressure and elevated LDL cholesterol, and helps raise the good (HDL) cholesterol. Onions contain dozens of powerful medicinal ingredients, including Sulphur compounds called thiosulfinates, which are thought to have strong anti-inflammatory effects and help with detoxification; phenolic acids, sterols, pectin, and volatile oils and vitamin C. Onions have also been shown to have strong antioxidant effects. They are a good source of the flavonoid quercitin, which is a potent antioxidant. Eating onions raw, pickled or cooked – are all beneficial in a cholesterol-busting diet.

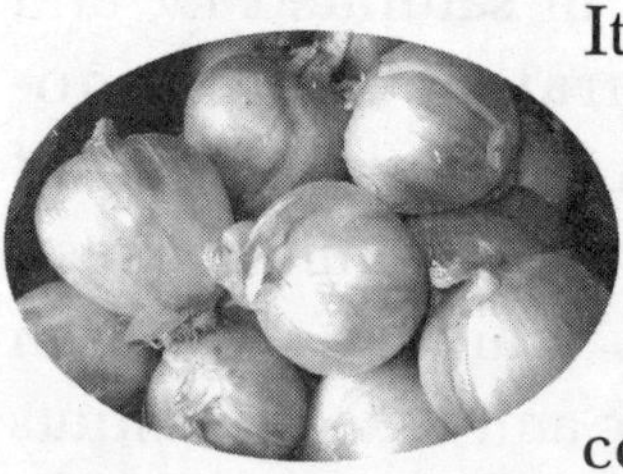

Pear

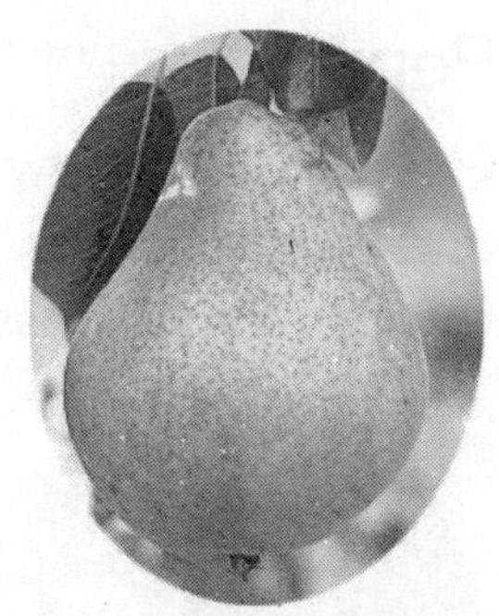

Pears contain lignin and pectin, fibres that bind to cholesterol while still in the intestine, preventing cholesterol from entering the bloodstream. Eating stewed pears for breakfast is recommended.

Peas

Dried peas, a small but nutritionally powerful member of the legume family, are a very good source of cholesterol-lowering soluble fibre, which forms a gel-like substance in the digestive tract that binds bile (which contains cholesterol) and carries it out of the body. Dried peas also provide minerals, B-vitamins, protein, and isoflavones (notably daidzein). Eaten boiled as salad or cooked in a curry, or even as sprouts, helps in lowering the dietary cholesterol.

Peppers

Green and yellow peppers are high in vitamin C and bioflavonoids. They also contain beta-carotene, folate and potassium. They possess powerful antioxidant properties. This means they protect against heart disease. Red peppers, along with vitamin C and bioflavonoids, are much higher in beta-carotene than green or yellow peppers and contain vitamin B6 as well as capsaicin, a natural painkiller. Experts consider red peppers to be especially beneficial against heart disease. The recommended way of eating peppers is more as raw salad than in cooked form.

Pineapple

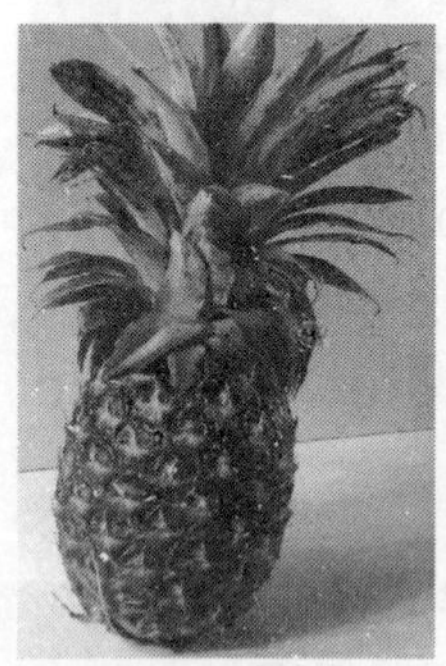

Pineapple is high in fibre and contains modest amounts of vitamin C, potassium and a unique digestive enzyme called bromelain. In addition, pineapple contains other micronutrients which some experts believe help disperse blood clots for increased heart protection. Pineapple fruit or juice is best taken in breakfast or as mid-morning snack.

Pomegranate

Pomegranates are proving to be the one of the most powerful antioxidants available. The cholesterol oxidation process, which creates atherosclerotic lesions that narrow arteries and result in heart disease, was slowed by as much as 40 percent when healthy subjects drank 2-3 ounces of pomegranate juice a day for two weeks. Further, the juice reduced the retention of LDL, the 'bad' cholesterol that after its oxidation aggregates and forms atherosclerotic lesions. It has also been found that the pomegranate juice slows down the damage caused by cholesterol, reduces blood pressure and more than doubles the levels of antioxidants in the blood. Pomegranate in any form should be consumed daily – fruit, juice, or powdered seeds as *chutney* or salad dressing.

Prunes

Prunes are dried plums, rich in iron and potassium. They are a very high-fibre food, containing more

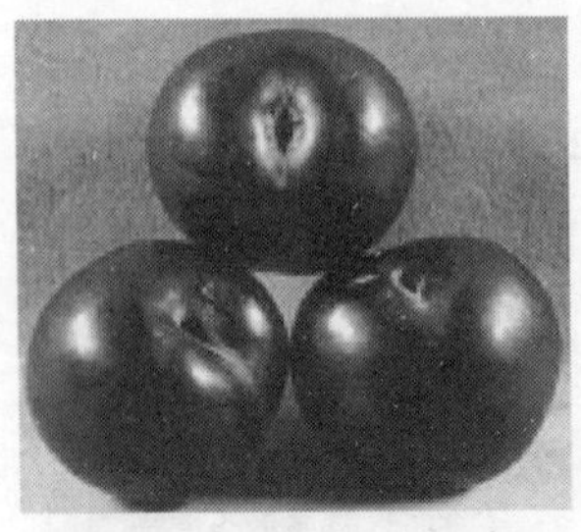

fibre than dried beans and most other fruits and vegetables. Over half of this fibre is of the soluble type that is linked to lowered blood-cholesterol levels. Prunes are also rich in beta-carotene and are a good source of B vitamins. Prunes are also a valuable food for anyone suffering from high blood pressure. Prunes can be consumed as such or be soaked in water and made into *chutney*.

Pumpkin

Pumpkin, especially the red one, is a rich source of beta-carotene and other carotenoids as well as the antioxidant vitamins C and E. It is also a good source of potassium. This makes it useful for lowering the cholesterol in the diet. Pumpkin seeds are a particularly good source of omega-3 fatty acid, and can be used in any food preparation, as they are bland and do not alter the taste while providing all the health benefits.

Red wine

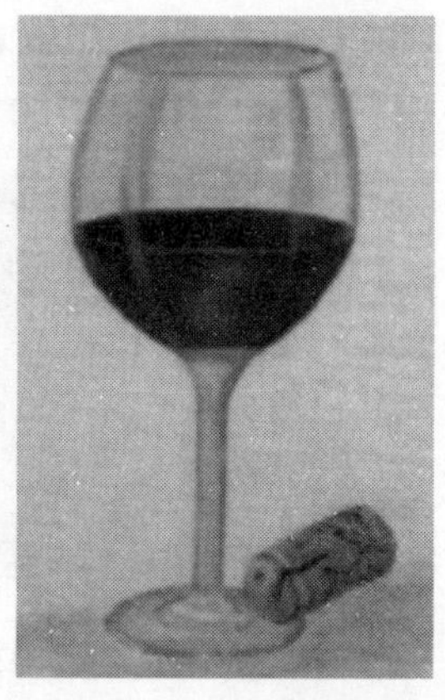

Studies indicate that red wine can raise HDL (good) cholesterol and prevent LDL (bad) cholesterol from forming. Red wine may help prevent blood clots and reduce the blood vessel damage caused by fat deposits. Another group of chemicals in red wine that is linked to the ability to lower cholesterol is called saponins. The association between red wine and decreased heart disease has also been attributed to resveratrol, a compound found in grapes, which acts as an antioxidant. But saponins could be just as important. Red wines contain about the same amount of saponin as they do resveratrol. But while resveratrol is thought to block cholesterol oxidation by its antioxidant action, saponins are believed to work by binding to and preventing the absorption of cholesterol.

Tomatoes

Tomatoes are high in the antioxidant vitamins beta-carotene, vitamin C and vitamin E, as well as the carotenoid lycopene. This means that tomatoes are helpful in preventing heart disease. Tomatoes

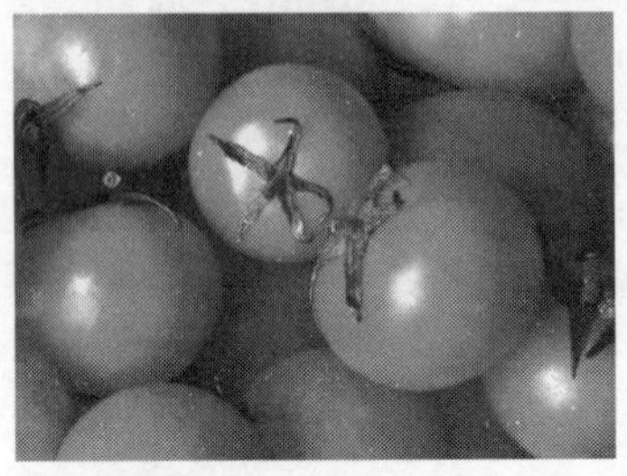

are also high in potassium but very low in sodium, which means they help to combat high blood pressure and fluid retention. Best eaten raw, tomatoes are very versatile and can be consumed as juice, soup, baked, grilled, or used in vegetables as curry.

Soya

Soya protein is the only vegetable protein that is complete with all eight essential amino acids. Soyabeans are a useful source of folate, vitamin B_3, vitamin B_6, vitamin E, magnesium, potassium, iron, copper, phosphorous and manganese. Research has shown that consuming an average of 47 grams of soya protein daily: decreased total cholesterol by 9.3%, decreased LDL-cholesterol by 12.9%, decreased triglycerides by 10.5% and increased HDL-cholesterol by 2.4%. The components of soya protein currently receiving the most attention are its bioactive components, in particular, isoflavones and phytochemicals. Phytochemicals in soyabeans protect the heart against oxidation, inhibit blood clot formation, function as antioxidants and also exert anti-inflammatory actions. Soyabean oil contains phytosterols, including beta-sitosterol, which helps to lower LDL (bad) cholesterol. Soya can be consumed as tofu, miso, nuggets, soyabean flour mixed with wheat flour and as regular beans.

Spices

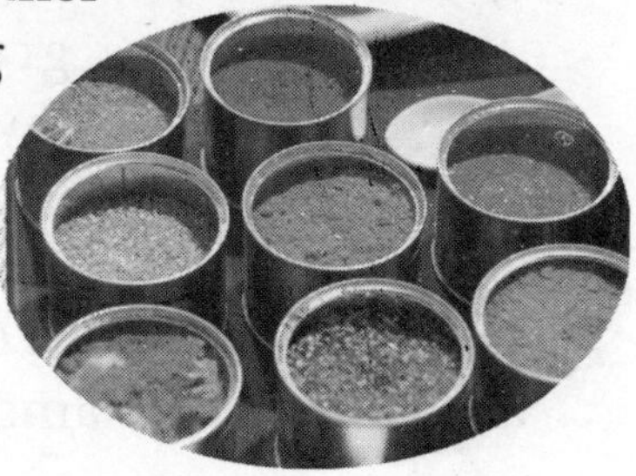

Most spices are potent antioxidants. Spices such as ginger and black pepper are added in diet to reduce cholesterol levels. **Ginger** contains two phytochemicals – gingerol, shogaol and an enzyme called protease, which aids digestion, helps lower cholesterol, and makes it a potent blood thinner. **Cayenne pepper** and other capsaicin-containing spices and peppers also boost heart health by reducing cholesterol and triglycerides. **Cinnamon** is packed with antioxidants, helping to control blood cholesterol and triglycerides, and has preventive powers against oxidative diseases such as atherosclerosis. **Turmeric** has antioxidants curcumin and curcuminoid with blood-thinning properties; fats get better digested, and cholesterol may be lowered. A substance in **black pepper** called piperine greatly increases the body's ability to benefit from spices, especially turmeric. It is advised to sprinkle crushed black pepper (or its powder) on the salads as much as possible. If not used in regular cooking, it is advised to use a pinch of cinnamon in at least one cup of tea in a day. Ginger should be consumed daily as cooked in any preparation or as pickled in limejuice.

Whole grains

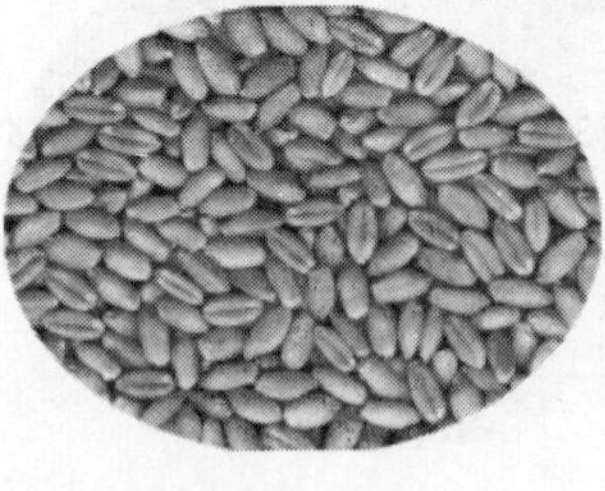

Whole grains like wheat, maize, oats, barley, millets, have three important parts: the outer bran layer, full of fibre, B vitamins, 50 to 80 percent of the grain's minerals, and phytochemicals; the large endosperm portion, full of complex carbohydrates, protein, and smaller amounts of B vitamins and the third part is the germ, full of B vitamins, vitamin E, trace minerals, and healthful unsaturated fats, phytochemicals and antioxidants. Eating three servings of whole grains per day helps decrease cholesterol levels, blood pressure and blood coagulation. It is advised to use the *atta* without removing its *chokar*. Corn or maize is rich in vitamins A and E, but should be used sparingly as it has a high fat content.

Yoghurt

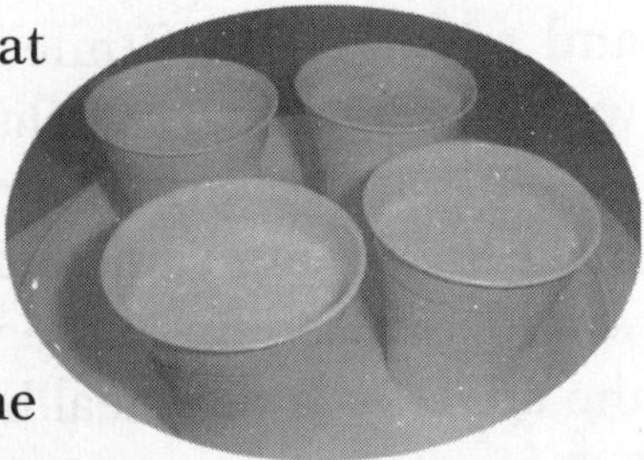

Some studies show that yoghurt can be helpful in lowering the cholesterol levels in the blood by decreasing the amount of cholesterol the body produces. There are a few studies that have shown that yoghurt can reduce the blood cholesterol. This may be because the live cultures in yoghurt can assimilate the cholesterol or because yoghurt binds bile acids, (which has also been shown to lower cholesterol), or both. Yoghurt is recommended for breakfast, mid-morning or lunch, but not for dinner.

PART IV

15-day Detox Plan

Our fore-fathers lived a healthier life than us, as they ate mostly fresh seasonal fruits and vegetables, did not drink aerated beverages much, did not use hydrogenated cooking medium much, and spent a lot of time in the natural sunlight, walking, climbing, socialising, lifting up things and in general moving around. Their bodies would make the required amount of cholesterol and excess would get used up in the various activities. This is the advantage of a healthy lifestyle.

If you find that your cholesterol levels are high, then begin with changing your diet first and then move on to improving your lifestyle. This is not easy, so it is advised to follow a plan, which can later be made a part of your daily routine or habit.

After much study of a number of alternative and traditional therapies and applying them practically in life, I came to certain conclusions and devised a comprehensive 15-day detox plan. It is a combination of diet including as many cholesterol-busting foods as possible, massage, *japa* and introspection. I have prescribed it to many and all reported positive results.

I would like to mention an interesting case study here, about a family all of whose members consult me on practically any and every health issue. The patriarch of this family suddenly had to be admitted in the hospital in a cardiac emergency. After stabilizing him, the doctors advised a bypass surgery for his heart. He had two major blockages in the blood vessels of his heart. But somehow he refused to be operated on, and reluctantly agreed for stenting of the blood vessels. As expected, his blood cholesterol levels were very high, blood sugar was hovering on the margin and he was hypertensive. Once he was discharged from the hospital, he called me for dietary advice. I prescribed my 15-day detox plan. It was wonderful to see him follow it religiously and more so to see that his blood profile came back to normal in six weeks. He became so enthusiastic about the plan, that I had to convince him to take a break for a couple of weeks from the detox regime. In the same family, his sister-in-law was discovered with very high blood cholesterol levels. The same plan was prescribed to her. But she could not handle the *japa* and introspection routine. The result was not satisfactory as there was only a marginal fall in the cholesterol levels. She was unable to de-stress, hence could not stop the cholesterol production in her body.

The point I am trying to make here is, that one needs to detox the body as well the mind to enjoy good health (and freedom from chronic disease).

I have already discussed the cholesterol-busting foods at length in the last chapter. The important thing now is for you to use them as much as possible in your daily diet. In the plan given below, barring the days of semi-fast, you are supposed to eat a normal diet following the prescription given earlier.

Day 1: *Semi fast:* Avoid salt, spices, non-vegetarian, all cereals and pulses. Have only fruits, vegetables, nuts, milk and milk products. Breakfast: fresh yoghurt (curd), banana and nuts; lunch: fresh cottage cheese and fresh vegetables (including potatoes) sauted lightly in oil with crushed black pepper; evening: fresh fruit; dinner: fresh vegetables only (add a little ginger), steamed or sauted and a cup of warm milk with honey. You may have herbal tea or lime-juice (*nimbu paani*) during the day. **This diet facilitates the exit of all forms of toxins accumulated in your body over a period of five days.** It also brings in a little discipline in your system.

Day 2: *Japa* the whole day: Choose any *mantra* as a *japa* – could be a single word, a phrase or a sentence. Repeat it throughout the day, in your mind. Even while you are working or traveling, you should do the *japa*. This exercise is a great help in channelising the positive energies in your body and disciplining your thoughts. **It's a stress buster, relaxing your mind without your realizing it, and hence reducing the stress-related cholesterol formation in your body.**

Day 3: *Oil massage:* Use warm til/olive/coconut oil. Massage your full body including head, preferably before going to bed. Have a warm bath the next morning. If it is not possible to do the massage in the night, you may do so in the morning, but a couple of hours before taking the warm bath. The massage should be done gently for at least thirty minutes, covering the entire body including fingers and toes. **The warm oil massage rejuvenates the blood supply, helping in breaking away of stored cholesterol, facilitating its exit from the body.**

Day 4: *Japa* the whole day, just like day 2.

Day 5: *Meditation and introspection:* Purification of mind to get rid of negative thoughts. Light a candle, sit comfortably on the floor, spine straight, look at the burning tip of the flame, absorb and shut your eyes till you visualize the flame. Visualize the flame in your mind glowing and purifying all thoughts. Move the flame to illuminate your entire body. Once you are satisfied that your entire body has been illuminated, open your eyes. Now, still sitting in front of the flame, think about the last five days in your life. Recall all the conversations you have had and all the emotions that you went through. Get rid of the negative emotions, forgiving those who were the cause of it. Accept your shortcomings and promise yourself that you would rectify them. Thank God for all the positive things that have been part of your life for the last five days. **This cycle is repeated every five days and along with the *japa,* helps you to relax consciously as well as sub-consciously, thereby reducing the demand and production of**

cholesterol by your body.

Repeat the entire five-day programme three times to complete 15 days, then give a week's gap and repeat again.

Cooking food

When cooking, use the following cooking methods more as they tend to produce lower saturated fat levels:

- ❖ Baking
- ❖ Steaming
- ❖ Broiling
- ❖ Microwave
- ❖ Poaching
- ❖ Grilling
- ❖ Roasting (use a rack so fat can drip away)
- ❖ Lightly stir-frying or sauté in small amounts of vegetable oil

Shopping for Food

❖ To keep your blood cholesterol level low, choose only the leanest meats, Choose chicken without skin or remove skin before eating. Remember, the white meat itself always contains less saturated fat than the red meat.

❖ Most fish are lower in saturated fat and cholesterol than meat or poultry.

❖ Since even the leanest meat, chicken, fish, and shellfish have some saturated fat and cholesterol; limit the total amount you eat to 150gms or less per day.

❖ **Meat substitutes:** Dry peas and beans and tofu (bean curd) are great meat substitutes that are high in fibre and low in saturated fat and cholesterol.

❖ Egg yolks are high in dietary cholesterol–each contains about 213 milligrams. So, egg yolks are to be limited to no more than 3 yolks per week, including those used in baked goods and processed foods. Egg whites have no cholesterol, and can be substituted for whole eggs in recipes – two egg whites to one whole egg.

❖ Like high fat meats, regular dairy foods that have fat – such as whole milk, cheese, and ice cream – are also high in saturated fat and cholesterol. Their intake should be limited to 2 to 3 servings per day of low-fat or non-fat dairy products or products made of skimmed milk. When looking for cheeses, go for the versions that are 'fat free,' 'reduced fat,' 'low fat,' or 'part skim.' The best would be to use cottage cheese or *paneer* made from skimmed milk.

❖ Choose liquid vegetable oils that are high in unsaturated fats – like corn, olive, peanut, safflower, sesame, soyabean, and sunflower oils.

❖ Buy margarine made with unsaturated liquid vegetable oils as soft tub or liquid margarine or vegetable oil spreads.

❖ Limit butter and cream. They are high in saturated fat and cholesterol.

- Buy light or non-fat mayonnaise and salad dressing instead of the regular kind. Avoid creamy white or cheese sauces.
- Choose whole grain breads as they have more fibre than white breads.
- Buy dry cereals, most are low in fat. Limit the high fat granola, muesli, and oat bran types that are made with coconut or coconut oil and nuts, which increases the saturated fat content. Add fat free milk or skimmed milk instead of whole milk to avoid saturated fat and cholesterol.
- Avoid confectionaries that are made with lots of saturated fat, mostly butter, eggs, and whole milk such as croissants, cakes, pastries, muffins, shortbread cookies, biscuits, cheese crackers, cream rolls, and doughnuts as all these are also high in cholesterol.

In A Nutshell

Follow the guidelines below to reduce your blood cholesterol and maintain a healthy lifestyle:

- ❖ Set a regular schedule of meal times and stick to it.
- ❖ Start your day with half a cup of water before having your bed-tea.
- ❖ Make breakfast your heaviest meal and dinner the lightest.
- ❖ Start your breakfast each day with an apple or pear, preferably stewed, skin included.
- ❖ Avoid eating until the previous meal is fully digested. Wait until you feel genuine hunger again.
- ❖ Eat until you are satisfied, not 'full.' Eat slowly and end the meal with a cup of any herbal tea. This helps to avoid over-eating.

- Drink half-a-cup of warm water before the meals, especially before lunch.
- Rest after getting back home from work for 15-20 mins in silence, eyes shut.
- Include fresh garlic in your diet. Saute one crushed garlic clove in a small amount of olive oil. Mix and eat with vegetables or dals.
- Squeeze fresh limejuice on your food just before eating.
- Sprinkle ground black pepper (*kali mirch*) in your meal before eating.
- Include pomegranate seeds, juice or powder (*anaardana*) in your diet on a regular basis. Pomegranate chutney could be eaten regularly.
- Use freshly ground cardamom (*ilaichi*), or the whole pod or seeds as you prefer, daily as desired in your food, tea, etc. Chewing two whole green cardamoms after every meal is recommended.
- Switch to whole grains. Avoid refined flours – do not remove bran (*chokar*) from the wheat flour (*atta*). Use more of whole pulses especially for dinner.

- Eat beans (soyabean or any other kind) at least three times a week.
- Eat more vegetables than other foods. Five servings (500gms) of vegetables every day is recommended.
- Choose whole fruit, skin included, instead of the juice.
- Eat foods that contain natural cholesterol busters, as much as possible every day. (Refer to the chapter on cholesterol-busting foods.)
- Have dinner at least two hours before sleeping and walk for at least 15-20 minutes after dinner.
- See to it that you get 6-8 hours of sleep daily.
- Follow the 15-day detox plan once in three months at least.

Bibliography

- AH Ensminger, ME Ensminger, JE Kondale, JRK Robson: *Foods & Nutrition Encyclopedia.*
- AH Ensminger, MK Ensminger: *Food for Health: A Nutrition Encyclopedia.*
- Francois Fortin: *The Visual Foods Encyclopedia.*
- Rebecca Wood: *The Whole Foods Encyclopedia.*
- Mary Meck Higgins: *Healthful Whole Grains.*
- WC Willett: *Intake of trans fatty acids and risk of coronary heart disease among women, Lancet 1993.*
- EH Ahrens: *Dietary fats and coronary heart disease: unfinished business. Lancet 1979.*
- R Beaglehole: *Cholesterol and mortality in New Zealand Maoris, BMJ 1980.*
- DJP Barker, C Osmond: *Diet and coronary heart disease in England and Wales during and after the Second World War, J Epidemiol Com Hlth.*
- PM McKeigne, GP Miller, MG Marmot: *Coronary heart disease in South Asians overseas: A review. J Clin Epidemiol, 1989.*

- ❖ V Ranskov: *Cholesterol lowering trials in coronary heart disease: frequency of citation and outcome. BMJ 1992.*
- ❖ JM Woodhill: *Low fat, low cholesterol in secondary prevention of coronary heart disease.*
- ❖ D Kritschevky, R Paoletti, WL Holmes: *Drugs, lipid metabolism and atherosclerosis.*
- ❖ Committee on Medical Aspects of Food. DHSS. 1984: *Diet and Cardiovascular Disease.*
- ❖ Washington DC, Dept. of Health, Education and Welfare, 1970: *The Framingham Diet Study: diet and the regulations of serum cholesterol.*